Feast
Without Fear

Food and the Delay, Don't Deny Lifestyle

Gin Stephens

DEDICATION

And a special message from me, Gin, to you, the reader

This book is dedicated to YOU: all of the dieters of the world, who have searched and searched for the "perfect" foods to eat. You know what I mean: that special, magical food plan that will lead to amazing weight loss and give you the body of a fitness model.

Does this one "perfect" diet even exist? Spoiler alert: NO.

My goal in writing this book is to teach you how to *Feast Without Fear*. You will learn how to choose foods that work best for your unique body, and why we are not all the same when it comes to foods that work well for us.

I am not here to be your health or medical guru. Instead, allow me to sit beside you in the role of friend: someone who has done the research for you, and is sharing the synopsis of it with you here, in this book.

The bad news is that you probably still won't have the body of a fitness model. Hey, maybe you will. (I don't.) But, even without that, the best news is that you will once again be free to enjoy the foods you love, free of the guilt that a lifetime of dieting has brought you.

Free to *Feast Without Fear*.

Also by Gin Stephens:

Delay, Don't Deny:
Living an Intermittent Fasting Lifestyle

Available through most online book and e-book retailers.

Visit
www.ginstephens.com
for blog posts and intermittent fasting success stories

Subscribe to *The Intermittent Fasting Podcast*!
Go to
www.ifpodcast.com
to learn more

Table of Contents

Foreword

Gin Stephens is one of the most uplifting and heartfelt authors I've had the pleasure to get to know. She and I connected privately after I joined her Facebook intermittent fasting support group, and I knew right away that Gin was someone who was genuine and kind. She has one of the most important qualities of every good teacher: never stop learning. As a doctor who is a fan of intermittent fasting, and an intermittent faster myself, I was immediately impressed with her knowledge and guidance on intermittent fasting. I admire her openness and willingness to connect to her readers, and how she encourages them to succeed.

Gin walks her talk and is a compassionate listener and communicator. She wrote her first book, *Delay, Don't Deny*, after losing 80 pounds and keeping it off for more than two years now. She created two very popular Facebook groups: *Delay, Don't Deny: Intermittent Fasting Support* and *One Meal a Day IF Lifestyle*. An avid believer in clean fasting and an active participant in these groups herself, she directs you back to the basic premise of intermittent fasting, while encouraging you to be in charge of what type of food plan you wish to follow. Although she has over 37,000+ followers in her Facebook support groups, Gin takes the time to give people individual attention. She is engaging, friendly, and well-educated, and if you'd like to get a taste of her Southern charm, you can hear her and her co-host, Melanie Avalon, as they answer readers' questions on their podcast: *The Intermittent Fasting Podcast*.

When you are an active participant in your online groups with a heart as big as Gin's, you want to see your readers succeed--and succeed they do! However, some come in looking for WHAT to eat, not just WHEN to eat. It's important to understand that when you are living an intermittent fasting lifestyle, your body and mind may be going through some amazing shifts behind the scenes: decreased pain and inflammation, cellular repair, reduced insulin resistance, autophagy, increase in human growth hormone, and an increase in neurogenesis and neuronal plasticity. But because of this, the more you have to heal, the longer it may take for you to see weight loss on the scale.

Gin recognizes, as do I, that people tend to hyper-focus and blame the food they are eating for the slow pace of their weight loss, rather than the fact that their body may be going through a series of adaptations and compensations. As a result, their body will shift between weight loss and healing and repair as it sees fit. Because of the dynamics of the body, people tend to fear eating the wrong types of food, and may eliminate entire food groups altogether, seeking a universal diet for weight loss. Sometimes, they will even give up before they reap the impressive benefits of intermittent fasting. *Feast Without Fear* will debunk the myths that you have to eliminate entire food groups in order to lose weight, or that you have to count calories, fat, or carb grams to succeed. It also will help you to understand that what works for me may not work for you.

As a Holistic Practitioner with over 18 years of experience, I can tell you for certain that Gin is right on-- there is no universal diet for weight loss. In my practice, I focus on food intolerances, leaky gut, autoimmune conditions, digestive health, chronic *dis-ease* and various inflammatory conditions. I practice functional medicine, which means I address the underlying cause of disease or dysfunction and focus on the health and healing of the whole person to bring them back into balance. I use a combination of lifestyle changes, mental and emotional counseling, essential oils, and plant-based medicine to bring patients' bodies back into an optimal state of health. I engage in a patient-and-practitioner therapeutic partnership, where we each play detective to successfully resolve their individual health challenges.

In my practice, each person is taught an individualized food plan based on their own biochemistry and how foods make them feel, and also based on how their bodies react. We work on optimizing their individual metabolisms by taking a look at the whole person: their food, sleep, exercise, stress level, and mental/emotional health. I teach my patients, as Gin does in *Feast Without Fear*, that food is information, not a math problem. I tell my patients that your body is more like a chemistry lab and less like a bank account.

There is nothing to fear on this journey. Your body wants to heal, it wants to thrive, it wants to perform optimally, and it wants to live at its ideal weight. As I do with patients in my private practice, *Feast Without Fear* will teach you to have a relationship with your body. First, you fast. Then, you feast. You wait, you listen, you live, you move, you pay attention to how you feel, you record feedback, and you begin again the following day. And the great part about this is, over time, as your body heals, the feedback changes, allowing you to eat more foods that may have bothered you in the past.

Now it's time to sit back, kick your feet up, and indulge in the deliciousness of experiencing a new relationship with food and your body. Allow Gin and her lighthearted humor to open your mind and touch your heart as she teaches you longevity lessons from around the world, information on how to heal your gut microbiome, how to tell what foods work for you, simple changes you can make today to experience vibrant health tomorrow, and helpful ways to take care of both your body and your mind. You'll also get to read some very inspiring success stories from people that never gave up and who will encourage you to keep pushing forward on your journey to health and permanent weight loss.

Bon Appetit, and Cheers to Feasting without Fear!

Dr. Kelley A. Kacergis, D.C., "Oil Doc"
Certified Intuitive Eating Counselor
Author of the e-program, *Are You In Your Driver's Seat?*
FB and Instagram: Ask Dr. Kel, Oil Docs

September 2017

Disclaimer

This book is not a substitute for medical advice. All information presented within this text is intended for motivational purposes. Any health, diet, or exercise advice shared here is the opinion of the author, and is not intended as medical diagnosis or treatment. If you think you have any type of medical condition, you must seek professional advice, even if you believe it may be due to diet, food, or exercise. You should always consult a qualified practitioner before using any dietary, exercise, or health advice from this text.

Locating links within the book

Throughout this book, I have provided you with links to research studies, websites, and articles. For readers who are using e-books, it's easy to click on a link and go straight to the source; however, for those of you who are reading the paperback version, the links aren't very useful.

Sure, you could very carefully type in each web address on any computer, but who wants to do that?!?!?! Not me!

For that reason, I have set up a webpage devoted to the links from the book. Visit:

http://www.feastwithoutfear.com/book-links.html

The links are organized by chapter and by page number (based on the corresponding pages in the paperback version of the book).

If you don't want to type in that whole link, you can simply visit:

http://www.feastwithoutfear.com/

and click on the tab called "Book Links."

Introduction

Why did I write this book?

I wrote my first book, *Delay, Don't Deny: Living an Intermittent Fasting Lifestyle,* in 2016, and released it anxiously on New Year's Eve. As 2017 dawned, people all around the world started to read my book, and as feedback rolled in, I realized that I had told a compelling story of hope for dieters everywhere, who were fed up with restrictive diets and the guilt surrounding every bite of food we put into our mouths.

In *Delay, Don't Deny*, I focused on the practice of intermittent fasting, and how changing WHEN you eat (but not WHAT you eat) could make a great deal of difference when it comes to weight loss and eventual weight maintenance. In that book, I explained how to apply the principles of intermittent fasting to create a flexible lifestyle designed around the way you want to live your life, celebrations and all. I also told my personal story of losing over 80 pounds after decades of struggling with my weight, and how I have been able to maintain the loss for over 2 years now, while eating all of the foods I love.

Yes, intermittent fasting changed my life, and nothing makes me happier than being a messenger of hope, sharing the practice of intermittent fasting (IF) with others. We may feel like early adopters in an "eat six times a day to rev up your metabolism" world, but I believe that the practice of IF is going to continue to spread until it becomes mainstream.

Through two Facebook support groups, I am watching thousands of members from six continents take back their health. (We are still waiting for the first member stationed in Antarctica…) The good news, we're learning together, is that we are not doomed to live our lives getting heavier and heavier, year after year. Where diets have failed us, this is a lifestyle that lets us live the lives we have always dreamed of, where we don't have to feel guilty every time we eat a meal, especially if we enjoy what we are eating. (Fun fact: as a society, we have trained ourselves to feel particularly guilty if a food is delicious. My goal is to change that!)

Since releasing my first book, I have watched many people as they have joyously transitioned to an intermittent fasting lifestyle with great success. It's incredible to hear stories from people expressing that for the first time, they can enjoy food without guilt. It's been life-changing for so many people.

Still—there are questions. Every day, people ask questions, such as: WHAT should I be eating? Are carbs okay? What about fat? Should I count calories? What about eating dessert? Can I have wine? How can I be sure I am getting enough protein?

In the support groups, people frequently post photos of their meals, and they are almost apologetic at times to be eating bread, or ice cream. Or—oh my gosh—a cheeseburger. Or pizza. Sometimes, someone will make a comment, such as "you would lose more weight if you cut out the ____" (insert your own idea of a "bad" food here). Of course, your idea of what is "bad" depends upon whatever sort of food rules you've internalized over the years.

In our support groups, we actually don't ascribe to any particular food dogmas or eating styles, other than the shared practice of intermittent fasting. When we tell newcomers to the group that they really can eat whatever they want, according to their dietary preferences and how foods make them feel, many don't believe us. They keep waiting for us to give them a food list or meal plan. When we don't, many people struggle with figuring out what to eat. So many of us have been on diets for decades, and we have therefore lost touch with even the most basic signals from our own bodies about what to eat and when to stop eating. And so, confusion about what to eat reigns supreme.

Even though we don't make specific food recommendations in our support groups, some people adopt an intermittent fasting lifestyle and find that contrary to the results of many other people, they don't have much success with weight loss, particularly at first. They struggle with the concept of eating "whatever they want," and some people realize that they don't lose weight until they do make some changes to what they are eating. I briefly touched upon this in the troubleshooting chapter of *Delay, Don't Deny*, but this new book should help people in this situation understand why their bodies may need something more than simply adopting an intermittent fasting lifestyle to see the best results. Yes, food quality does matter!

While it's true that up until now I haven't made any food recommendations in the support groups, that is about to change, here in this book. The goal of this book is to cut through the confusion and highlight what foods are most likely to promote vibrant health for most of us, and why.

To understand why we are all so confused, think about this: over the years, the message about what foods we should (or shouldn't) eat has gotten more and more muddled. As an illustration, think about the changing perception of eggs over the decades. Eggs have been an important food in the human diet for thousands of years, but suddenly one day everyone was concerned about cholesterol, and eggs were seen as the enemy. Of course, you could throw away the yolk and eat the whites only, but that left you with a rubbery tasteless heap of egg whites. So sad. You could dress it up with some equally rubbery fat-free cheese if you wanted to go totally nuts. (*Raise your hand if you ever ate an egg white omelet made with fat free cheese. Now, smack yourself in the forehead to remove that image from your brain, forever. Your taste buds will thank you.*) I remember how the egg industry tried to recover with an ad campaign for *The Incredible, Edible Egg*, but the damage done by the anti-cholesterol and low-fat movement continued for years—and even to this very day, some people continue to worry that the egg yolk is somehow bad for us. Other people consider the egg yolk to be the part of the egg with the most nutrients, and so they embrace the yolk.

So: should we eat eggs, yolk and all? Are eggs good for us, or are they slowly killing us? How do we know? Hopefully, after reading this book, you will feel more confident about the answers to these questions.

Before taking any advice from me, you probably wonder who I am. How am I qualified to write a book about health or food in the first place? Time for me to come clean. I am not a nutritionist, I have not been to medical school, and I don't have any medical credentials. Instead, I have a bachelor's degree in elementary education, a master's degree in science education, and a doctorate in gifted education.

While my elementary students do call me Dr. Stephens, I am not a medical professional. That's one reason that I won't give you medical advice in this book, and please understand that you shouldn't take anything I am saying as an actual health recommendation from me to you. Always check with your doctor for health concerns or specific questions that you may have, particularly before making any changes in prescribed medications.

I am not a doctor, nor do I play one on TV (sorry, kids…everyone my age and older gets that joke); but I am a teacher. I have been in the classroom with students for 28 years. As a teacher, it has been my life's work to learn things and then teach those things to others.

In my work as a writer, I am still doing what I have always done as a teacher: I am learning as much as I can about the topic at hand, and then presenting it to you. I am going to provide you with links directly to the original sources, so you can check these things out for yourself. Do

12

your own research! Verify everything I tell you, and then dig even deeper into the science.

We no longer live in an era where all of the knowledge is locked up by scholars and held tight in the colleges and universities, only to be shared with the privileged few. In today's information age, anything we want to learn about is literally at our fingertips 24 hours a day. This is both a blessing and a curse, as I am sure you know. For any topic you can imagine, you can type a few words into your search bar and immediately be bombarded with more information than you could ever hope to process, much of it contradictory. In fact, if you want to have some fun, go to your internet browser and type this in the search bar: *water will kill you*. I found 120,000,000 results. Are you scared of water yet? Apparently, you should be. You're welcome.

As I have already said, food, and how we should eat, is one of the most confusing topics out there. Fortunately, we are learning more and more about how the body works every year. Scientists are surprised at some of the new discoveries, particularly in the area of the gut microbiome. I plan to share some of these discoveries with you in this book. My goal is to present it to you in a way that piques your interest and leads you to do further research. Some of the information I present may, indeed, be contradictory to what you believe to be true. Heck, doctors can't even agree on this stuff, so why shouldn't WE be confused?

One more thing about me, and why I felt compelled to write this book: I have always been interested in food. I can still remember where I was sitting in my 4th grade classroom when we had lessons on the basic food groups and what our bodies needed for us to be healthy. It was fascinating to me. Sometimes, we were asked to keep food logs that we were supposed to bring in so we could analyze if our diet was healthy or not. (I remember doing this task more than once over the years. Maybe teachers only had one nutrition lesson plan back in the seventies.)

Funny story—I always faked my food log—every time. Even then, I knew that there was a great deal of judgement surrounding food. Instead of writing down what I really ate, which was probably along the lines of Beef-a-roni or a TV dinner (some of you are too young to know what that means, but it involved the oven and about 45 minutes of waiting before the foil-covered meal would be ready), I would make up some meal that sounded more virtuous. I knew that the "right" foods were important and made us "better" people. Perfection through a falsified food log in elementary school. Sad.

If a school assignment allowed us to do something with food, I was all over it. As an example, once in 6th grade, we were assigned a project on the human body. We had to create some sort of 3-D model as a part of the assignment. I made cookies in the shape of body parts, and we all ate them in class after my presentation. Delicious or macabre? You decide.

In my early teens, I was active in 4-H. You may not be familiar with 4-H, but it is a club that has its roots in rural communities throughout America. One of my favorite 4-H competitions involved demonstrating a task in front of an audience and a panel of judges. I remember that one year I demonstrated how to make omelets (yolks and all...the horrors). The next year, my project was about how to make crepes. I brought in a crepe maker and everything. Yes, I loved to cook! Even though I had a Beef-a-roni and TV dinner palate, as I already mentioned, I loved what I could do with food.

The fascination continued. In high school, I took a class on computer programming. The programming language was *Basic* (no, really—that is what it was called), and we saved our work on cassette tapes that plugged into the monstrous computers we used. As our final project, we were tasked with creating a computer program of some sort. Guess what mine was about? Ding, ding, ding! Yes, it was about food. At the age of 15, when I was a slim teenager, I created a calorie counting program. You could decide on your calorie count for the day, and then enter a combination of meals and snacks to ensure that you stayed under your limit. If you still had calories "left over" after planning your meal, the program gave you a message that said, "Congratulations! You have saved enough calories to enjoy a cookie!" or something like that. My computer science teacher loved it.

Yes, as you can see, I have always been obsessed with food in one way or another. As I got older, the obsession with food for the sake of food itself turned into an obsession with dieting and weight loss. Even when I was a lean teenager, I focused on dieting for my calorie counting computer program. I didn't need to diet, but it seemed like the thing to do at the time. This fixation on dieting continued for decades.

I told my whole crazy dieting story in *Delay, Don't Deny*, and many people have confessed that my saga reminded them of their own dietary struggles. Over the years, I read every book released on how to eat. Most books contradicted other books that I had read, and it became more and more confusing. Is it any wonder that I gave up and just resigned myself to getting fatter and fatter?

I am so grateful that I discovered intermittent fasting in 2009! Even though it took me until 2014 to adopt it as my lifestyle, once I did, I finally lost the obsession with what to eat, and I was able to effortlessly lose the excess weight that I needed to lose. It felt like a miracle.

Now that I have learned how to maintain a healthy weight, I can once again focus on my love of food. Cooking is now my hobby, and I enjoy preparing delicious foods for my family and myself.

A funny thing happened, though. The freer I became with food, the more I learned to listen to my body, and the more I paid attention to how foods made me feel. Now that I have "permission" to eat whatever I want, the foods I want have changed dramatically. I have learned what foods make me feel vibrantly healthy, and I have also learned what foods don't work well for my body. I don't need an "expert" to tell me what to eat: my body makes it clear to me. If that sounds nutty, rest assured that you absolutely can regain the ability to listen to YOUR body, just as I have.

In this book, I will talk a lot about food. What should **YOU** eat? What should **I** eat? Is it the same for everyone? When do individual differences come into play? What is "good"? What is "bad"? And how do we know for sure, when the experts can't even agree?

What the heck should we eat? And why?

This book may challenge some of your ideas about "good" and "bad" foods. Choosing what foods to eat often feels overly complex, and yet it may be much simpler than you believe. There are certain types of foods that fit into an overall health-promoting template of sorts, and we can design our personal eating plans around this template.

While reading this book you're going to realize that your body is incredibly unique, and there are many reasons why this is true. You'll learn that any "one-size-fits-all" dietary recommendations can't take your individuality into account.

As you learn about these individual differences, you'll be better equipped to understand why some foods work better for you than others, and also why your plate won't look exactly like my plate.

What does it mean to *Feast Without Fear?*

It means that:

- You should not fear any real foods that people have eaten for hundreds or thousands of years. While that doesn't mean that all foods will work equally well for your unique body, it's empowering to realize that you don't need to be afraid of real food.

- Your body doesn't respond exactly the same way to foods as my body, because we each have unique characteristics that come into play.

- You have the power to figure out what foods work for you, and once you do, you can ignore all of the conflicting advice out there. Your body has a way of communicating over time what foods make you feel best. You'll learn to trust the messages that your body is sending you.

Now, it's time for us to learn how to *Feast Without Fear!*

Chapter 1

Food fear in the modern era

If you go back in time, food was simple. Our early ancestors gathered and hunted based on what was around, and once they found food, they ate it. Starting around 9,500 B.C., people all around the world began domesticating both plants and animals, and the era of agriculture was born. People grew and raised what was suited for their climate, and just as our hunter/gatherer ancestors...when they had food, they ate it. All around the world, different civilizations developed their own harvest festivals to enjoy the bounty from the earth. Food was celebrated, and people truly did *Feast Without Fear*.

Pretend that you could go back in time to one of these ancient celebratory feasts. Assuming you could communicate with them (why not, since we are time traveling), imagine having a debate with someone about whether they should be eating so many carbs, or if they really think that extra helping of mutton is a good idea. Your words would be absolutely meaningless to them, and you would probably have to worry about being burned at the stake if you started talking about the calories, vitamins, or macronutrients in their foods.

Yes, back then, food was simple. The main concerns centered around making sure there was enough to eat, as famines could cause total devastation to their communities. Abundance was seen as a blessing, and food was something to be enjoyed.

Now, we no longer fear a lack of food. Our modern era is faced with problems related to overabundance rather than lack, and the obesity crisis is one result of the current food climate. Instead of waiting for the harvest festival to feast, we can head over to the local buffet restaurant and feast three times a day if we want to, with snacks in between.

Spoiler alert: we were never meant to eat this way.

These days, we all know that we need to eat less food, but that's easier said than done. We also wonder what exactly we should be eating. As the endless debates rage on, we are getting one consistent message about food, no matter where you turn:

Everything you want to eat will kill you.

We seem to have entered some sort of alternate universe where there are so many theories about what food is good and what food is bad that we are almost afraid to eat. Name a food…any food…and I can show you someone's recommendation to avoid it for health purposes.

If you are on social media, I'm sure you see friends sharing article after article about what we should either be eating or avoiding. These articles come with sensational headlines designed to draw you in, so you will read it and see what "latest" scientific discovery you need to be concerned about. As an example, I will call the summer of 2017 "The Summer of the Coconut Oil Battles." Based on a new set of dietary guidelines released by the American Heart Association, people were sharing articles saying that coconut oil is the worst thing you could ingest due to the high saturated fat content, while others were frantically posting rebuttals stating that there is no need to worry about the saturated fat found in coconut oil, and the other articles were all wrong. The anti-coconut oil experts cited scientific studies and so did the pro-coconut oil experts. After reading both sides, you were probably more confused than ever about coconut oil, not knowing who to believe. Or, you may have decided to ignore whichever perspective didn't align with your own dietary belief system, which is what many people do.

Is it true that everything you want to eat will kill you? Let's analyze all of the food groups and see if it is true. I am going to think back...WAY back...to when I was a student in elementary school in the 1970s, sitting in that same 4th grade classroom I mentioned in the introduction. This was before the days of the Food Pyramid or "My Plate." No, we kept it simple, and all we had were the 4 basic food groups: Milk (which included all dairy products), Breads and Cereals (all grains fit into this group), Fruits and Vegetables, and Meat (even though we called it the "meat" group, it also included all high protein foods such as fish, beans, and nuts).

Here's the shocking information that you have been waiting for: now, thanks to the latest medical research, we have learned that each of the 4 food groups is, indeed, trying to kill you. It's true! Let me tell you how, one by one.

Let's start with the milk group. Milk? Are you kidding? Dairy products are only safe for baby cows. You are probably drinking cow mucus. Gross. You shouldn't have ANY dairy in your diet, period. Bye-bye, cheese. Bye-bye, ice cream. Dairy is completely off the menu.

On to the next food group. Breads and cereals? They are the absolute worst. You may not know this, but all grains are literally killing you as we speak. Even though they have been a foundation of the human diet for thousands of years, we have recently learned that humans aren't meant to eat grains. They are destroying your intestinal tract and it's surprising that you can even read this, due to the detrimental effects of grains on your brain. Gluten? Pure poison. If you aren't gluten free, you should be.

Finally, a food group we can all agree on as healthy: fruits and vegetables. Surely those are safe, right? Ha! No. Nobody needs carbs. Carbs make you fat. Didn't you know

20

that? Fruits and vegetables are high carb, just in case no one ever told you. Carbs=BAD. Fruits are actually full of fructose, which was invented by Satan himself.

What's left to eat? Meat? Oh, come on. Everyone knows that you shouldn't eat a lot of meat, especially red meat. It's full of cholesterol and fat. No meat for you. Nuts also have way too much fat and too many calories. At least you can eat fish, right? Not so fast. Fish are full of contaminants such as mercury. You definitely don't want to eat fish. And poultry? Have you ever seen how they are raised? Salmonella awaits you in every bite.

There is actually one other food group, and we called it the "other" group. All "fun" foods fall into that category, such as candy, desserts, dressings, oils, butter, and the like. Bad news: you already know all of those fun and delicious foods will kill you, so there is no need for me to elaborate. No fun foods for you, and if you eat one, please feel an appropriate amount of guilt. It's the right thing to do.

So, what's left to eat? Sorry. There's nothing left. Everything will kill you. You're just going to have to live on water.

Wait…remember our earlier internet search, where I found 120,000,000 results about how water will kill you? There's even more bad news about water…unless it comes in the right kind of container, or has just the right pH, guess what? If you said that your water has many ways that it wants to kill you, congratulations. You're right. At least 120,000,000 of them.

I hope you realize this discussion of the dangers from every food group has been tongue-in-cheek. Of course, your foods are not trying to kill you.

Foods nourish our bodies. Just as our great-great-great grandparents knew, there is a great deal of value in having a well-balanced diet, including a wide variety of foods from all food groups. They may not have understood why, but they knew it to be true. How have we lost sight of this wisdom? In this book, we will learn how to re-train our brains so that we are able to *Feast Without Fear*!

The message of this book is this: you really do have room in your diet for all food groups. You can even eat foods from the "other" group.

Here's a funny side note. I am picturing readers who are now thoroughly upset by that last paragraph. Some people are going to be mad that I just recommended dairy products, while others can't believe that I just cavalierly told you that it's okay to eat grains. Or carbs. Or fat. That's because there is SO MUCH emotion tied into what we eat. It's become like a religion for many. And, just like religions, there are factions and sides.

While researching for this book, I read and watched everything I could put my hands (and eyes) on. Some of it is, frankly, depressing.

If you want to worry even more about the state of our society, forget about politics: go to the internet and read scathing reviews of those who promote opposing dietary recommendations. I have seen mean-spirited videos that "fat shame" certain dietary experts. There are entire websites devoted to tearing down the "other side" and presenting their particular side as the One True Way to Salvation.

Every one of these websites has videos showcasing reputable doctors (most of whom have written a book) who present medical study after study illustrating why their church, I mean diet, is the best one for all of mankind, and explaining to you why the other side is just plain going to Hell, I mean getting sicker and sicker.

If you want to really be confused, watch a documentary produced by vegans, and then watch a video produced by someone who promotes a ketogenic or low carb diet, high in animal fat. How can each side have doctors saying the exact opposite things as the other side? How can they all have studies that show that their diets are the best, while the other side has studies showing that their (completely opposite) diets are the best?

After viewing the compelling evidence from both sides, you might be so scared that you're willing to try to live on the most dangerous of all substances: the water I am now so worried about. (Sarcasm alert: I'm not really worried about water. Just in case you wondered.)

As a society, how did we get this way? I blame it on:

- **The media**, who love to sensationalize everything. Every time a scientist releases a new study about food or nutrition, the media gleefully reports it. These days, if we aren't in a constant state of panic about something, they aren't doing their jobs.

- **Diet gurus**, who write diet books that claim to have all of the answers you need spelled out precisely within the pages. Every new diet promises to solve your specific health and weight problems. Never mind that every book contradicts another book out there. Never mind that another diet guru has a blog post calling this diet guru a complete quack. How can they both be right, when they are completely opposite in their recommendations? And, aren't they both doctors? Shouldn't they both understand science the same way? Can they both be right and both be wrong at the same time?

- **Our personal doctors**, who haven't been adequately trained on nutrition. You can't blame them, because according to a report put out by the National Institutes of Health in 2008, *"The results of our recent survey show that most medical schools are not providing adequate nutrition instruction."* To read that report in more detail, including how

they came to their conclusions, go to:
https://www.ncbi.nlm.nih.gov/pmc/articles/PMC2430660/

- **Ourselves!** Sorry, but we have to share some of the blame. We have read book after book, listening to expert after expert. As a result, we have jumped on so many bandwagons over the years that we can no longer make simple decisions about what to eat without being afraid that we are messing everything up with each bite. The more we look for the "perfect" way to eat, the harder it is to enjoy a meal.

The result is that as we become more and more confused about what to eat, we may end up throwing up our hands and giving up completely. I know that's what I did for a number of years. Everything is bad for me, huh? I guess I'll just eat this large pizza and drink a soda, because at least it's delicious.

The good news is that we can filter through the confusion and figure out what foods are good for us. The better news is that our bodies are smart enough to give us feedback about what we are eating, once we learn to listen.

In the chapters ahead, I am going to talk about how the longest-living people in the world eat, and it may surprise you. We are going to learn about the individuality of our own bodies, and why certain foods may work for me but not for you, and vice versa. It turns out: we are not all exactly the same, and our bodies do not process foods the same way, no matter what diet guru #1 or diet guru #2 may claim. Finally, we will talk about what happens if you can't tolerate certain foods that you would really like to enjoy again. In addition to what we eat, I am going to mention some other lessons we can learn from the longest living people in the world. We can make a few lifestyle changes that enhance our lives in other ways, unrelated to what we put on our plates. It turns out health is more holistic in nature, and not just about what we eat.

Overall, this book will provide a template for what may be the "ideal" way to eat in a broad sense, with recommendations of how to adjust this template to suit your unique body. After reading this book, you should understand why this is true. Also, once you understand this important concept, you will be better equipped to ignore any "one-size-fits-all" dietary strategies, that don't actually "fit all," because they can't and don't take your individuality into account.

My number one goal is to teach you how to *Feast Without Fear*!

Before we get into specifics about foods, though, let's talk about my favorite dietary strategy of all: intermittent fasting! If you want to *Feast Without Fear*, one of the best ways to do it is to start with an intermittent fasting plan that suits your lifestyle.

Chapter 2

Intermittent fasting: A primer

If you somehow stumbled onto this book without first reading *Delay, Don't Deny*, you may not know much about intermittent fasting. I'm going to discuss the basics in this chapter, but to really understand how and why to live an intermittent fasting lifestyle, you need to read *Delay, Don't Deny*. This single chapter can't go into the depth that I went into in the first book. Even if you are an experienced intermittent faster, I still recommend that you read my first book, if you haven't read it yet. Why? Here's an example: because of the conflicting information out there, there were several mistakes that I made inadvertently over the years, and fasting wasn't as effective as it could be until I understood the science and made some changes to my regimen. All of those topics are discussed in detail in the first book.

If you have read *Delay, Don't Deny*, you'll still want to read this chapter, because I am going to be sharing some information that may be new to you. I'm getting a bit more science-y in this book.

So, what is intermittent fasting? Even if you eat three meals a day plus snacks, like most people in our modern society, you are a faster, whether you realize it or not. We all fast while we sleep, and we wake up every morning in the fasted state. Most intermittent fasters simply extend that fasted state throughout the day rather than eating a traditional breakfast in the morning. Just like everyone else, we break-fast, but it may be when most people are having their dinner. "Breakfast" literally means "break the fast."

We all do it, just at different times of the day. For me, break-fast, which I usually eat in the evening, really is the most important meal of the day!

During most of the day we fast, and when we eat, that is called our "eating window." There are many different approaches to intermittent fasting, and the most common eating windows vary between one and eight hours a day.

To illustrate how this looks, let's say someone follows an intermittent fasting lifestyle with a 4-hour daily eating window. Since a day has 24 hours, twenty hours of each day would be spent fasting (including the time you are asleep), and all of your eating for the day would take place during the consecutive 4-hour eating window that you choose.

Here's how I apply this into my life. Every morning, I wake up and start the day with black coffee. After my coffee, I switch over to water and unflavored sparkling water until I am ready to eat. I usually open my eating window at some point between 4:00 and 5:00 pm with a snack of some type. A couple of hours later, I prepare dinner for my family, and I eat with them. After dinner, I will often have a glass of wine or a dessert of some type. Overall, my eating window lasts for somewhere between three to five hours most days.

For those who have never heard of intermittent fasting, this may seem bizarre or even possibly dangerous. What?!?!?! You go most of the day without eating? Don't you have headaches? Don't you collapse from lack of food? How do you have energy to do day-to-day tasks? Many intermittent fasters have gotten the speeches from well-meaning friends and family members:

"You are putting yourself in starvation mode!"

"Everyone knows that breakfast is the most important meal of the day!"

"You must eat 6 small meals per day to keep your metabolism from shutting down!"

Not one of those statements is true, even though we have probably all heard them. You aren't going to go into starvation mode, and your metabolism will be just fine. In fact, your metabolism may end up running at a higher level than ever before. Stay tuned. But first, let's talk about the many health benefits related to this lifestyle.

While most of us begin living an intermittent fasting (IF) lifestyle with the goal of losing weight, IF is about so much more than just weight management. Even if you never lost a pound, I am convinced that IF is one of the healthiest things you can do for your body. Instead of damaging your body or your metabolism, IF has the potential to improve your health in many ways. I actually like to call it the health plan with a side effect of weight loss.

It's such a powerful wellness approach that my husband lives an intermittent fasting lifestyle now, and it's strictly for the health benefits. Unlike many of us, he has never needed to lose weight, and he still fits into the same pants he wore at our wedding back in 1991 (annoying, right?) Based on what I have shared with him about the power of IF, he has decided to follow an 8-hour eating window most days, which gives him at least 16 hours of daily fasting. During the work week, he eats within an 8-hour eating window each day, although he is somewhat more flexible on the weekend when he wants to be.

So—what's so special about IF that an always-slim man would adopt it as his lifestyle? It's actually pretty exciting, and it is why I will be an intermittent faster for the rest of my life. Time to dive into the science behind IF!

Over the past year, the biggest news in the intermittent fasting world was without a doubt the announcement of the 2016 Nobel Prize in Medicine. As written in the press release, Yoshinori Ohsumi "discovered and elucidated mechanisms underlying *autophagy*, a fundamental process for degrading and recycling cellular components." What stimulates autophagy in humans, you may ask? Fasting! Let's take a few minutes to understand what autophagy is, and why we want to encourage it to occur in our bodies.

Here's a link to a scientific article that explains autophagy. It's called *Autophagy Fights Diseases Through Cellular Self-Digestion*, and it was published in 2008.

(Note: remember that whenever I discuss any study, journal article, or website, I am going to give you a link to it within the text. Many people read books on electronic devices now, and it's a lot easier to click on the link right within the text vs. having to turn to a reference list in the back of the chapter or the back of the book. I want you to have the information right at your fingertips, so I will always provide it for you. You can go straight to the source and see what it says, rather than just take my word for it. If you are reading this in traditional paperback book form, go to www.feastwithoutfear.com to find ALL of the links from the book organized by page number, for your convenience.)

https://www.ncbi.nlm.nih.gov/pmc/articles/PMC2670399/

When reading that publication, as with any, start with the abstract to get an overall idea of what the paper is about. In this case, you see that the paper explains the basics of autophagy at the cellular level, and what that means to us.

In this particular paper, some of the most important information is found in Figure 3. If you click on the link for Figure 3 within the study, you can expand the illustration to see some of the diseases and conditions autophagy addresses within our bodies at the cellular level. It's a pretty exciting list: cancer, heart disease, liver disease, infections, autoimmune conditions, and even diseases related to aging. We all know friends and family members who are affected by these conditions, and the thought that we may be able to prevent them by something as simple as fasting is thrilling.

So, how does autophagy work within the body, and when does it occur? There's a lot of debate about when autophagy actually starts in humans (even among the various physicians who promote the practice of intermittent fasting). You'll hear all sorts of varying theories, in fact; but based on all of the evidence (and opinions) I've read, this is the picture that emerges. As always, remember that I am not a biochemist or physician, and these are extremely complex processes that are still being explored and understood by scientists. It's also possible that a few years from now, our understanding might change, based on new research.

Some of the clues can be found in this journal article. It's called *Autophagy and Metabolism*, and it was released in 2010:

https://www.ncbi.nlm.nih.gov/pmc/articles/PMC3010857/

As with the other paper, start with the abstract. You'll notice that the paper describes autophagy as a process the body uses "in starvation." That makes the fasted state sound alarming, as we equate starvation with negative outcomes. Try not to let the word scare you. When you are an intermittent faster, you aren't in danger of starving. This term is simply another way of describing the fasted state. In this article, starvation=the fasted state, in contrast to the fed state, which is when you are eating.

Take a look at Figure 3 in the second paper to see a diagram showing how autophagy works within the body. (It's a coincidence that both papers have the good stuff in Figure 3.) When you read the caption for Figure 3, you see that these scientists estimate that the processes of autophagy ramp up when our bodies have depleted our body's glycogen stores. (Glycogen is quick energy our bodies stick away in predominately our liver and our muscles, and it's the first place our bodies will turn for energy when we are fasting.) Once we burn through our stored glycogen, our bodies have to find a new source for energy, and this is when we can most efficiently begin to tap into our fat stores.

Tapping into our fat stores is the goal of any diet plan, and fasting helps us do it in a way that a traditional "diet" could never do. When we finally tap into our fat stores, we begin to make ketone bodies through a process called ketogenesis, and the state we call "ketosis" occurs (not to be confused with ketoacidosis). Once this happens, it appears that the process of autophagy ramps up. Assuming that this estimate is accurate, that means that when we live an intermittent fasting lifestyle, we will have periods of the day--every day--where our bodies are focused on cellular housekeeping. While fasting, I love visualizing my cells hard at work taking out the cellular trash, keeping me healthy at the cellular level. Hooray for autophagy!

One question many people have involves just how long it takes to deplete your glycogen stores, and it causes a lot of confusion in the intermittent fasting community. Let's assume for the sake of simplicity that you have 2,000 calories worth of glycogen stored in your body, as that is a number you'll see thrown around as an average. If you start fasting right now, it might take you 48 hours to deplete all of that glycogen (though it could take more or less time, because there are many factors at play). For that reason, many people claim that you won't ever be able to get to the magical state of ketosis (and therefore, you won't experience increased autophagy) unless you fast for at least 48 hours straight. Some people also believe that you can only get into ketosis if you are eating a low carb or ketogenic diet during your eating window. Fortunately for us, that isn't true.

This is a complicated concept for many people, even me, and I am going to explain it in what may be an over-simplified way (remember, I am not a doctor, and so my explanation is coming from a layperson's perspective), but it should still give you an idea of how it is possible to reach a state of ketosis during your fasting time, even if you eat carbs in your eating window (which I most certainly do).

Assume that you're a brand new intermittent faster, and that you start with full glycogen stores on day 1. This means that your body has plenty of quick energy packed away for you to tap into as needed. On that first day, you'll burn part of the way through those stores, until it is time for your eating window. When you eat, your body will partially refill your glycogen stores with some of the energy from that meal, but your glycogen stores will not fully refill. The next day, the process repeats. The good news is this: every day, if you are fasting correctly and for a long enough period of time, you should burn more of your stored glycogen during the fast than you add back after eating. Every day, your glycogen stores will go down further than they were the day before. Eventually, one day during the fast you will have depleted your glycogen sufficiently to switch over to the state of ketosis.

How long does this take? I can't tell you, because it depends on too many individual factors, such as what you eat, how much you eat, and your metabolic state. Many people find that the state of ketosis is one of the most enjoyable parts of an intermittent fasting lifestyle. Once you reach this state, most people have a lot of energy and mental clarity, which is nice. You lose the afternoon slump many of us are used to when following a typical three-meals-a-day eating pattern. The down side is that you may notice a strange metallic taste in your mouth, or others may report that you have bad breath. Take that as a badge of honor, and try not to breathe too closely on anyone you love.

If you want to deplete your glycogen stores quickly, you may choose to start off with a 48 hour fast to kick things off. It's not necessary, though, and if you are patient, intermittent fasting will get you there over time. You don't need to stress over exactly when it is happening: trust the process, and understand that your body knows what to do. You may feel tired and sluggish (and HANGRY) during the adjustment period, but if you stick with it, it's so much better on the other side. I have suggestions in *Delay, Don't Deny* for how to get through this initial adjustment period.

Now, back to the second paper on autophagy. There's a lot of interesting information in this second paper, but scroll down to the section that explains how autophagy plays a role in the regulation of metabolism. This section explains first how the process of autophagy is used in the body to clear out fat from the liver, which is a really good thing. A fatty liver is associated with both insulin resistance and metabolic syndrome, which are frequently seen in obesity. The very last paragraph of that section leads to some more exciting news: apparently, insulin resistance in mice can be reversed through the process of autophagy. We aren't mice, but many scientists believe that this process works the same way in humans.

The section on the metabolic impact of increased autophagy is also interesting. The authors note that as we age, both our body's overall energy expenditure and rate of autophagy generally decline. That means that we may experience weight gain (due to lowered energy expenditure, or a lowered metabolism) and also increased effects of aging (due to decreased autophagy). We've all heard of this, and most of us think it's inevitable: you'll gain weight as you get older, right? Maybe not! When we are fasting, we experience increased autophagy on a daily basis. Might increased autophagy also increase energy expenditure in the body as we age? The authors don't come right out and say it, but the connection may be there.

Yes, understanding the role autophagy plays in our health is exciting. Our bodies have a built-in mechanism for fighting both diseases and the aging process, and all we have to do is take a break from eating constantly. It's the easiest (and laziest) approach to health imaginable. Instead of actively doing something, you just stop doing something: don't eat constantly, all day long, like most of the world seems to do these days. Genius!

Instead of warning us about dangers related to skipping meals, anyone who understands autophagy should encourage us to start skipping meals, for the health benefits alone.

Notice that I led with the amazing health benefits of intermittent fasting, because I want you to have that first and foremost in your mind. IF is healthy, with powerful anti-cancer, anti-inflammatory, and anti-aging benefits, just to name a few. As I already said, even if you never lose a pound, it is worth doing for the health benefits alone.

But—is it crashing your metabolism, as critics warn? Despite the health benefits, are you putting yourself in danger of slowing your metabolic rate, resulting in long-term damage to your metabolism, and eventual weight regain? Fortunately, the answer appears to be no.

Another study, called *The Cardiovascular, Metabolic and Hormonal Changes Accompanying Acute Starvation in Men and Women,* is often cited by intermittent fasting experts, and I included it in *Delay, Don't Deny*, as well. It's such an important study that I am including it here, too:

https://www.ncbi.nlm.nih.gov/pubmed/8172872

Unfortunately, even though I have read the full study, all I can link here is the abstract, so you won't be able to read the full study for yourself from this link. It's always just a bit risky to go by the abstract only, because the details are within the full papers. Regardless, we can read some very exciting information about metabolic rate within the abstract itself. According to the authors, the participants' resting metabolic rates *increased* after 36 hours of fasting. In addition, the participants saw no metabolic slowing from baseline, even through the 72nd hour of fasting. (It is interesting to note that the metabolic rate increased from the 12-hour point to the 36-hour point, but did slightly decline again from the 36-hour point to the 72-hour point. The overall metabolic rate at 72 hours was still slightly higher than that noted at the 12-hour point.)

The authors attribute the increased metabolic rate to the processes of gluconeogenesis and ketogenesis, which we read about in the paper on autophagy and metabolism. Apparently, the body uses a lot of energy to carry out these

34

processes, which may be the key to the slight metabolic boost we experience.

Remember: you should not be alarmed by the use of the word "starvation," which the authors use to describe the fasted state. In this particular study, they are referring to periods of intermittent fasting from 12-72 hours in length. No one ever starved to death in 12-72 hours. (Though my cat often thinks he is going to starve to death if he can see the bottom of the cat food bowl. My cat is not an intermittent faster, as you can tell.)

The take-away from that study is this: scientists found that metabolic rate increased slightly between 12-72 hours of fasting (just as the previous article hinted in its discussion of autophagy and energy expenditure). Metabolic shutdown? Clearly not! On the contrary, metabolic rate went UP!

To summarize what we have learned so far in this chapter:

1. Fasting may just be one of the healthiest things you can do for your body. It stimulates autophagy, which is how your body naturally takes out the cellular trash. The more I read about it, the more I believe that it's one of the most powerful things you can do for your health. In fact, if you told me I could go back to eating all day long and still maintain my 80+ pound weight loss, I wouldn't do it. I prefer to experience the health benefits that go along with increased cellular autophagy.

2. Intermittent fasting appears to be great for your body metabolically. Rather than slowing your metabolism, which we find in diets that promote long-term calorie restriction, IF has metabolic benefits that you miss out on when you follow the typical diet plans that have you eating frequently throughout the day. The key to the success of intermittent fasting lies in the processes your body experiences during the fasting period.

After reading this, you should realize that intermittent fasting is not some radical new fad diet that is here today, and gone tomorrow. Think about it: fasting is actually an ancient practice that is seen all around the world and in every major religion. The good news is that in intermittent fasting, you are not being asked to go 40 days and 40 nights without food: with most intermittent fasting plans, you are eating until you are satisfied every day, and most people find that it's a lot more enjoyable than trying to eat tiny unsatisfying meals spread throughout the day. Once you adjust, it's actually easier than typical diet plans. This is one of those things that most people don't believe until they try it for themselves.

Now that you understand how many benefits are associated with IF, you should be confident that it is a healthy and desirable lifestyle choice. If you haven't already experienced intermittent fasting for yourself, you probably want to know how to begin. Fortunately, I have a whole book devoted to that topic. If you haven't already done so, I encourage you to read my first book: *Delay, Don't Deny: Living an Intermittent Fasting Lifestyle*. In it, you'll learn about several different approaches to intermittent fasting, and how to develop a plan that suits your own lifestyle.

One of the most important principles to understand about intermittent fasting is that you want to keep your insulin as low as possible during the fasted state. This is all explained in detail in *Delay, Don't Deny*, but I want to mention it here because it is important. As a quick summary, insulin is a hormone in our bodies that is related to fat storage, and one popular theory is that when insulin is high, our bodies have a difficult time accessing our fat stores. In contrast, when we keep our insulin levels low, our bodies are better able to access our stored fat, which is essential for ketosis (because we want our bodies to produce ketones from our fat stores). I want you to think back to figure 3, linked from the second study on autophagy I mentioned in this chapter (I'm putting it here again for your convenience):

Ketogenesis, or the production of ketone bodies for energy, is a key feature that occurs during fat burning. Our goal during the fast is to keep our body happily burning fat for fuel, rather than risk stopping these processes. If you ingest something during the fast that causes a substantial insulin release in your body, your body will stop burning fat and insulin will do the job it is designed to do: move glucose from your blood into storage. That is the exact opposite of what we want to have happen.

As I said, this is all explained in *Delay, Don't Deny*, so make sure to read it to learn why and how to fast effectively so you reap maximum benefits. I made several rookie mistakes which made fasting more difficult and less effective before I understood the science.

Since we now understand that one of the goals of the fasting period is to keep insulin as low as possible so we can access fat stores and experience all of the benefits related to ketosis and autophagy, you may have questions about what you should consume in your eating window. Which foods should you eat? Is there, in fact, one "best" way to eat?

I decided it was time to answer the question that many people ask: when we feast, does it matter what we eat?

Chapter 3

In search of the "perfect" diet

When I decided to write a second book about food and eating, I made it my goal to figure out once and for all just what we should all be eating. This should be easy, right? With all of the information out there, it should be possible to figure this out. It's 2017. We eat. We know stuff. How hard can this be?

I started by thinking of food at its most basic level. Foods that we eat are made primarily of three "macronutrients." These are carbohydrates, proteins, and fats. At various times, each has taken a turn in the spotlight as either the hero or the evil villain of our diet, even protein. (To illustrate this point, there is one diet book named *Protein Power: The High Protein/Low Carbohydrate Way to Lose Weight, Feel Fit, and Boost your Health — in Just Weeks!* and another called *Proteinaholic: How Our Obsession with Meat is Killing Us and What We Can Do About It.* Both are written by doctors, yet have completely different recommendations about protein's place in our diets.)

Looking over the diet trends of the past few decades, a few stick out as most influential.

I thought back to the 1990s, when dietary fat was the enemy. We were all told to eliminate as much fat as we could from our diets, and we would all be healthier and slim. Experts explained that our bodies are great at turning dietary fat into body fat, and the more fat you eat, the more fat you will store on your body. That makes a lot of sense theoretically when you think about it. Unfortunately, many of us missed the point. Rather than choosing foods that were naturally low in fat, such as high-quality fruits, vegetables, and whole grains, we instead turned to low-fat "food-like products" (anyone else remember eating an entire package of fat free cookies? Why not? It's FAT FREE!) One problem is that those low-fat foods, particularly the overly-processed variety, are not very satisfying. Also, highly processed foods are not good for us (for many reasons), and the fat-free replacement versions of foods have little in common with real foods. Most fat-free and low-fat foods are filled with chemicals to simulate the mouth-feel of the fat that they are replacing. Yuck.

After the low-fat era, we moved to the low-carb period. Fat was back on our plates, but carbs were out. We had a new dietary villain. The low-carb premise is based on the science of insulin as a storage hormone. As I mentioned in the last chapter, the insulin hypothesis states that if you have a lot of insulin circulating throughout your body, you aren't going to be great at burning fat, though you will be great at storing fat. Because we know that carbohydrates (most particularly the highly refined versions) tend to raise insulin levels the most, it logically follows that when we eat foods that don't stimulate much of an insulin release, we won't have as much fat-storing going on. Low carb diets promise that if we simply restrict carbohydrates, we can eat as much as we want of other foods, including protein and fat, and we will effortlessly lose weight. There is one big problem with that, however, and it is the fact that protein also stimulates insulin release. Oops.

This information was a big surprise to me. I remember reading Dr. Atkins' books, where he described a metabolic advantage that would give us easy weight loss with an unlimited amount of food, and all we had to do was limit carbs below a specific threshold. That never worked for me, and now I understand part of the reason why. When I followed a low carb eating plan, I swapped out carbs and added in lots of protein. I ate high protein snacks all day long, in fact. Cheese and sausage! Meatballs! Bacon! However, if you look at something called The Insulin Index, you will see some surprising results related to protein. Here is a link to a paper published in 2009, called *Food Insulin Index: Physiologic Basis for Predicting Insulin Demand Evoked by Composite Meals:*

http://ajcn.nutrition.org/content/90/4/986.full.pdf

Within this paper, you can see the FII, or "Food Insulin Index" score, for a variety of foods. A beef steak (FII=51) actually elicits a higher insulin response than white pasta (FII=40). No, that is not a typo. Even raisins (FII=42) promote a smaller insulin response than a beef steak. Who would have thought that white pasta and raisins would raise insulin less than a beef steak? Not Dr. Atkins, that's for sure. If your only goal is lowering your insulin response to foods, you'd be better off having some corn (FII=53) than having a piece of fish (FII=59). Surprised? Me, too. (Note: I found the FII of fish in a different article, called *An Insulin Index of Foods: the Insulin Demand Generated by 1000-kJ Portions of Common Foods*, which is from 1997. I am unable to link this study here, because it isn't available online. The FII numbers used in other studies all originate from this original 1997 study, as far as I can tell.)

Of course, the body is complex, and we know it's not as simple as only measuring the insulin response to an isolated food. Even though protein raises insulin levels, it also stimulates glucagon, which is a counter-regulatory hormone. We know that the glycemic response also factors into how our bodies process specific foods (more about the individuality of the glycemic response in another chapter—stay tuned!) The point is, however, that it's never as simple as it appears to be on the basis of any one measurement, whether we are discussing the FII or the glycemic index. Much like a Facebook relationship status, "It's complicated." Even so, if your goal is reducing insulin, which the low-carbohydrate diets recommend, it's clearly more complex than simply limiting carbs.

So, the low-fat recommendations didn't work for most of us long term, and neither did the low-carb and high protein diets. In recent years, we have moved in another direction in the diet arena. The latest dietary trend includes once again eschewing carbohydrates while also moderating consumption of protein. What's left if you avoid carbs and don't eat as much protein? That leaves us with fat. Unlike the low-carb diets of the past, the new turbocharged version, called the ketogenic diet, suggests that we would all be healthier if we eat mostly fat, with very few carbs and moderate amounts of protein. A ketogenic diet recommends that you get 65-75% (or more, depending on which guidelines you follow) of your daily intake from fat. As with intermittent fasting, eating foods high in fat also stimulates the process of ketosis, which is the basis of the word "keto"-genic. If ketosis is good, we must want it 24/7! Let's have ketosis that never ends!

You can see that with the ketogenic diet, we have circled exactly 180 degrees from the low-fat food recommendations of earlier decades. Everything the low-fat diet plans warned about, the ketogenic diets encourage us to eat without abandon. Fat is suddenly where it's at.

Low fat. Low carb. Ketogenic. As I pondered the "ideal human diet," I thought back to these three main dietary trends of the past decades. Each makes sense theoretically, right? You probably know someone who has had great results on a low-fat plan, and someone else who swears by a low-carb diet. Many people have amazing results from a ketogenic approach. Certainly, one of these plans has to be the overall winner, and therefore reign supreme as the one we should all follow. The only question is which one. Is it low fat? Low carb? Ketogenic? I decided that I wouldn't stop until I had figured it out. This was easier said than done, as you can imagine.

I pulled out every book I had that focused on diet plans. (And I had a LOT of them.) I located the studies that were referenced in the back (the ones that most people don't read). I watched documentaries. I combed through PubMed (PubMed is the online database of the US National Library of Medicine, and it includes all scientific studies you might be interested in...and plenty more that you would actually not be interested in).

My goal was to see where the research took me. I threw out all preconceived notions and looked for a common thread. Could I find evidence to support a low-fat diet as the ultimate diet for humans? Would low-carb be the winner, after all? What about the ketogenic plan...is it the diet savior for all that it's touted to be?

The more studies I read, the more confusing it became. I found studies that seemed to contradict other studies. Some of the studies were done on rats and mice. Others were conducted with few participants, over a very short duration. Many studies focused on isolated dietary components, when, in fact, most foods (and the meals we create out of these foods) aren't made of one single macronutrient or component.

As I looked deeper and deeper, I found that every single style of eating had studies that both supported it and refuted it, at least on a surface level.

When we want to find out what is the "best" diet for us to eat, it makes sense to start where I did...looking to the scientists and their isolated studies for the answers. But— there are limitations with scientific studies. The ones conducted on rodents or other animals may have results that are not transferrable to humans, and the ones conducted on humans may be flawed, short term, or include too few people to draw meaningful conclusions.

Let's take a few minutes to talk about the state of scientific research. How did science bring us to the point where we are all utterly confused about food?

Chapter 4

In science we trust?

Scientific studies: we can't get enough of them! I've already mentioned a good number of them in this book, along with links to the studies themselves. We learn a lot from scientific research when it is done well. But first, let's talk about a few of the problems with scientific studies, and why we can't take everything we read at face value.

To help you understand this, I want to take you to elementary school, and start with the scientific method at its most basic. You may start reading this chapter and think, why is this here? Trust me: it's important to understand the basics of scientific inquiry in order to analyze and critique any studies you may come across. So, let's have a science lesson! Stay with me here, because later I am going to connect this to the bigger picture of scientific research in general.

Let's see how this works in the world of 4th grade science. To do an experiment, you first must come up with a question that you would like to answer. Paper airplane experiments are a classic in the world of 4th grade, so let's say little Johnny wants to do a science experiment about paper airplanes.

Johnny knows what he wants to do. He comes up to me with his question: which type of paper makes the best paper airplane? Sounds like a great experiment, right? Not quite. Immediately, I ask Johnny to think about the wording. What does he mean by the word "best"? Is it the one you like the best? The one that is easiest to fly? The one that goes the farthest? The one that is most durable?

Now little Johnny is a little irritated with me, because he has to go back to the drawing board. Eventually, he comes up with a better question: does the type of paper used in construction affect how far a paper airplane will fly?

After coming up with a good question, you generally develop a hypothesis, which is what you believe will happen. Johnny believes he knows what type of paper is best, so he records his hypothesis.

Next, you need to design the experiment itself, to test the hypothesis. This is where it gets tricky. One of the most important parts of designing a good experiment has to do with carefully identifying and controlling your variables. First of all, you have to figure out the manipulated variable that you want to test: that's the one thing you are changing in your experiment. Next, you have the responding variable, which is what you are measuring (your outcome). Finally, you have the controlled variables, and those are the all of the things you must keep the same throughout your experiment.

Within Johnny's question, you can see both the manipulated variable and the responding variable. The one thing he is changing is the type of paper (the manipulated variable), and he will be measuring how far the planes will go (the responding variable). Nothing could be easier, right? Is Johnny ready to do his experiment?

Not yet. And Johnny is going to be irritated again, because it's time to talk about controlling the variables in his experiment. He has to make sure that everything is the same except for the one thing he is changing, which is the type of paper he's using. You can't just start folding paper airplanes and throwing them, because there are many variables to consider. (Johnny, of course, wants to go straight to the airplane throwing step. Sorry, Johnny.)

44

What are some of the things that need to be controlled in this experiment? First, the paper should all be the same size, and that's harder than it sounds. If you are in a typical classroom, you'll find notebook paper, construction paper, and copy/printer paper. Did you know that all three types of paper are slightly different sizes? If we just start making paper airplanes out of these convenient types of paper, then they will all be slightly different sizes. Suddenly, we have an experiment that is about different *types* of paper AND different *sizes* of paper. When we look at our results at the end of the experiment, we will know which airplane went farthest, but we won't know why. Was it the *paper type* or the *size difference* that made the plane fly farthest? Because we don't want to have two things that are different, we need to make sure that we are choosing paper that is the same size. So, we can control that variable by cutting the different types of paper so that they are all exactly the same size.

This is usually the point when Johnny starts trying different airplane folds, and decides that he wants each plane to have a slightly different design, because it's a lot of fun to make different types of planes.

Sorry, Johnny, you can't do that, either. Every plane needs to be the same design. While it may be boring, it's important. Otherwise, you have added yet another variable, and that is airplane design. No, in order to see if the type of paper makes a difference in how far the airplane will go, you have to use the same design each time.

Now Johnny has 3 different airplanes that are made from the same size paper, and they are all folded the same way. He is ready to start throwing these planes.

Or is he? Sorry, Johnny. No.

Imagine you are throwing a paper airplane a bunch of times. Will you throw it the same way each time? No, of course not. At the beginning, you will be new to airplane throwing. Maybe your technique isn't good. Somewhere in the middle of the throwing session, you will find your airplane-throwing groove, and it'll be easier to throw it successfully. After a while, though, your arm will get tired, and your technique will suffer. In order to truly make sure we are launching the plane the same way each time, we need to take the human element out of it entirely. Johnny needs to design an airplane launcher, so that every launch will be consistent.

Once Johnny gets his launcher designed, it's finally time to start the experiment. He needs to make sure to have several trials for each of his paper-types, and when he is done, he will calculate the average for each type of paper to analyze his results.

While Johnny is doing his experiment, there are still some things he will need to watch out for. Occasionally, something will go wrong and he'll get an unexpected result, like if another student jumps in front of the plane after it is launched. (This is surprisingly common in the world of 4th grade plane experiments, and is pretty much a guarantee, in fact.) Should he record that result, or toss it out and try again? It's important for him to keep good records that explain exactly what went on during the experiment, particularly anything that might affect the overall results.

One other thing that Johnny has to watch out for is experimenter bias. Remember: back at the very beginning of the process, Johnny developed a hypothesis. Because he believes that one type of paper will make the best airplane, he needs to make sure that he isn't somehow steering the results to match his preconceived ideas. This is a lot harder to do than you realize, actually. (If you don't believe me, study quantum physics, which teaches that the very act of observing something changes results. Once you study quantum physics, you will start to question the very existence of matter, so I try not to think about it too hard. I just can't. Sorry, quantum physicists. You are on your own.)

Back to Johnny. Finally, he will be done. He will calculate his averages, analyze the data, and determine if his hypothesis was correct. (It isn't surprising that most of the time, the initial hypothesis is shown to be correct. Is this because students are great at making hypotheses, or because of experimenter bias subtly affecting results?)

It's usually at this point that some girl in the class will come up and tell Johnny that his results aren't valid because the plane he made out of construction paper is heavier than the others, which is an additional variable he forgot to control for. She is technically right, and now we see how difficult it is to design a good scientific experiment.

I hope you stuck with me through all of this, because I am trying to make a point. If it is this hard to design a good experiment about paper airplanes, how much harder is it to design an experiment that deals with *people*? How do we even begin to control variables in experimental studies with different people? It's impossible to do so perfectly, actually. There are too many variables that come into play. Did the subjects follow the guidelines correctly? If it is a diet study, are they cheating on the diet in secret? (It is at this point that I recall my own falsified diet logs from back in my elementary school days, where I faked everything I was eating just so my teacher would think I was somehow better than I actually was...)

Even if you keep all subjects in a controlled setting and feed them all of their meals while you are watching them, there are still going to be problems. For one thing, any dietary study should be conducted over a sufficient period of time in order to actually judge what is happening. We all know that long term results are going to be different than short term results, no matter what dietary strategy we are studying. How many people are going to be able to spend a long period of time living in a controlled laboratory setting? Not very many.

I read a lot of scientific studies, as you can imagine. Often, I can see the flaws right in the abstract, which is the summary of the study (and the only part that many people read). As an example, I recently read the abstract of a study where three dietary approaches were compared, with the goal of determining which was superior for weight loss and overall markers of health. Each of the three test diets included different types of foods from the others. Two of the test diets involved the same number of calories (they were both described as "restricted calorie," within certain dietary constraints), while the third test diet allowed subjects to eat as much as they wanted within another set of dietary constraints (it was described as a "non-restricted calorie" diet). Hopefully, you already see the most obvious flaw in this study. How in the world can we compare three diets when the variables were so different? Can we determine anything of value when we compare two "restricted calorie" diets to one that is "non-restricted"? Clearly, we can't, and I am pretty sure my 4th graders would understand that. This was also a study that depended upon the subjects following the dietary guidelines on their own, away from the researchers. Did they? Well, they said they did. Just like I claimed I ate carrots, when I was really eating Beef-a-roni.

Dr. John Ioannadis, a scientist affiliated with Stanford University, published a paper in 2005 called *Why Most Published Research Findings are False*. You can read his paper here in its entirety:

https://www.ncbi.nlm.nih.gov/pmc/articles/PMC1182327/

What??? Most published research findings are false??? That's a pretty bold claim, but highly important to understand. If you go to the link I just shared, first read the summary at beginning of the article to get an overall idea of Dr. Ioannadis' thoughts. As you get into the article, some of it will probably be confusing to you as a layperson, but go to the section on "Corollaries" to see his analyses about what makes a study less likely to be reliable. These include things such as small sample sizes, financial and other interests of the researchers, and "hot" new fields of study.

Do I agree with him that "most" research findings are false? Not really. But, I do think that it shows us that we can't simply take any scientific study at face value without understanding certain things about how the studies were conducted. It encourages us to be skeptical and to question what we read.

If you want to do more reading about some of the problems that go along with scientific research, an eye-opening book about this topic was just released (2017) by Richard Harris. It's called *Rigor Mortis: How Sloppy Science Creates Worthless Cures, Crushes Hope, and Wastes Billions*.

Harris's book is about issues found throughout the biomedical sciences. As you dig into this book, you'll find discussion about one of the problems with this type of research: replication, or repeatability. A good study should be repeatable, which means that when we repeat any scientific experiment, we should get the same results. If you think back to our paper airplane experiment, this means we should consistently find that the same type of paper makes the airplane fly the farthest. If we get a different result each time we repeat the experiment, that's a problem.

As an example, I read a study that said that only about one third of psychological studies could be replicated. Oh, the irony of using a study about studies to prove a point…

One of the main problems with scientific research appears to be related to data analysis. According to the authors of *False-Positive Psychology: Undisclosed Flexibility in Data Collection and Analysis Allows Presenting Anything as Significant*, one of the problems is that data can be manipulated to give an impression that results are statistically significant, when they really are not. To read about their findings in detail, click on this link:

http://journals.sagepub.com/doi/pdf/10.1177/0956 797611417632

While this article focuses on the field of psychology, the problem of inappropriate data analysis seems to apply across the whole biomedical field. Harris's book goes into it in greater detail, if you are interested in specifics.

So, what can we do? How can we know that what we are reading is true? Can we rely on any scientific studies at all? What is the takeaway from this chapter? Are we doomed???

I believe the message is this: we need to approach all scientific studies with a bit of skepticism. Don't ever take the headline as truth. Dig in. Read the study for yourself, if possible, and look at the whole study rather than the abstract whenever you can. Be critical of the study design. Remember what you learned about variables from our paper airplane experiment example. Did researchers keep everything the same, other than the one variable they were testing? How large was the sample size? Did the researchers have any financial interests in the outcome of the study?

About that last point: it's important to for you to know that much of the research in the United States is funded by companies. Do you think the breakfast cereal companies would have a financial interest in a study about breakfast being the most important meal of the day? Funny how that happens, isn't it?

If you are interested in learning more about how deep the financial interests of various corporations may go, you can take a look at an article from the Journal of the American Medical Association. The article, written by Marion Nestle, is called *Corporate Funding of Food and Nutrition Research: Science or Marketing?* This link takes you to the first page only, though I have read the full 2-page article (you need to access it through a university library or subscription to see the whole thing, which is common with many scientific journals):

http://jamanetwork.com/journals/jamainternalmedicine/article-abstract/2471609

Dr. Nestle examined 76 studies conducted from March-October of 2015 that were funded by industry. According to Nestle, 70 of the 76 studies "reported results favorable to the sponsor's interests." Pretty convenient, hmmm? Is that just a coincidence?

There is one more thing that I want you to understand about how scientific studies are used. It is common for authors to use (and misuse) scientific evidence to support a position. Whenever you are reading a book (or article) written in support of a particular dietary strategy, the author is going to cherry-pick research studies that support his or her position and ignore any studies that may cast doubt. (In my reading of diet books, I often notice that an author will claim within the text that a study proves one thing, but when you actually go to the study and read it, that is not what it says...at all. They don't think you will take the time to read the studies themselves, apparently.) Also notice that an author is able to identify all of the flaws in conflicting studies cited by those with opposing viewpoints, but is blind to any flaws in his supporting evidence. This is called confirmation bias, and it's human nature.

Well, I'm a human, too. So, as you read anything I write, please go straight to the articles themselves, and also don't hesitate to critique the study design or look for flaws. I won't mind, because I didn't design or conduct the studies myself. Always question. This is what I teach my elementary students, and it's what I want to teach you to do, as well. Anytime I cite a study, you also want to verify that what I am telling you is actually what the study or article reports, and that I have interpreted it correctly.

Now that you have read this chapter, you may be even more confused. If you can't completely trust research studies, what can you trust? Well, for one thing, you can trust how you feel. If you feel better eating a certain way, then it's probably right for you. If you find that your health is improving in ways you can measure, and this continues long term, you can bet that this particular approach is probably a great match for your body. Our bodies are

amazing, and they give us many clues once we learn to listen. If, however, you continue to feel worse and worse over time, or health markers are moving in the wrong direction, that is usually a sign that something isn't working for you. I will talk about this in more detail later.

So, what can we do? Is there any way to scientifically assess the human diet to see what is "best"? Has science failed us? In some ways, maybe. I actually think we have been looking in the wrong place for many of the answers we seek.

We've been looking in the science lab, when the answers we are looking for may not be found there at all. The answers may be found somewhere else entirely. Actually, I believe there is a blueprint out there for us to follow. Based on my research, I believe the answers lie in two places: we can look at the dietary and lifestyle habits of the longest-living people on earth, and we can also look deep within our own selves, into our deep, dark gut microbiomes. When we do, we will notice that the diets that seem to keep humans alive the longest also feed our gut microbiomes the best.

Is this just a coincidence? I don't believe that it is. To figure out what to eat, let's take a look at what we can learn from these two very different, but linked, places: the world outside of ourselves, and the world within us.

To begin, let's see what we can learn about food from some of the longest-living and healthiest people in the world.

Chapter 5

Longevity lessons from around the world

If we want to *Feast Without Fear*, we can learn a lot from the people who actually live this way.

According to Dan Buettner, there are five places in our modern-day world where we can decipher the secrets of a long and healthy life. Buettner has worked with scientist Michel Poulain and the National Geographic Society for over 10 years to find and study the longest living populations on earth. To conduct their groundbreaking research, a team of scientists from various disciplines traveled the world to see what these five different populations have in common, and what lessons we might take from their lifestyles. Their work was partially funded by the U.S. National Institute on Aging, and what they found gives us many insights into health and longevity.

Overall, the type of research they conducted involves studying a population over time, and then drawing conclusions based on findings. Of course, we can't necessarily determine *causation* from these types of studies, but we can discover *correlations*. Correlations are patterns that seem to be associated with certain outcomes. We can't prove that one factor caused the other, but we see that they tend to be related in some way.

Buettner and his team spent a great deal of time among the various populations they were studying, and based on what they found, they named these five longevity hot-spots the "Blue Zones." They include:

- Ikaria, Greece;
- Sardinia, Italy;
- Okinawa, Japan;
- The Nicoya Peninsula in Costa Rica; and
- Loma Linda, California.

In all five areas, they found people living into their 90s and even past the century mark. These people aren't just living a longer life; they are healthy and thriving. While we can learn a lot from their diets, they also teach us many things about how to enjoy life. They are active: rather than exercising for the sake of exercise, they all move purposefully as they go about their daily tasks. They also have a strong sense of community, share food with those they love, and live a low-stress lifestyle when compared to Americans or others around the world who live a hectic modern lifestyle.

Unlike many of us who follow a typical Western diet, these people don't count a single calorie. They couldn't tell you the ratio of carbohydrates, protein, or fat in their meals if you asked them. They are the longest living people on the planet, but they don't feel stress about what they eat or worry about what foods are on their plates. They eat. They enjoy their lives. They celebrate together.

I highly recommend that you read Buettner's original article, "The Secrets of Long Life", which was published in *National Geographic* in 2005. It can be accessed in its entirety in a free pdf form through the bluezones.com website. Here is a link to it:

https://bluezones.com/wp-content/uploads/2015/01/Nat_Geo_LongevityF.pdf

The Blue Zones website (https://bluezones.com) is full of fantastic information about how the people from these five different populations live, and also includes lessons we can apply to our lives. As always, I encourage you to go to the source to read for yourself. The Blue Zones website has many articles to read and videos to watch, and you could spend hours browsing around and taking it all in.

In addition to the original article and the information found on the website, Buettner has written several books that I highly recommend: *The Blue Zones: 9 Lessons for Living Longer from the People Who've Lived the Longest; Thrive;* and *The Blue Zones Solution.* That last one includes all of the dietary recommendations in one place, and gives overall suggestions about how we can apply lessons from the Blue Zones to determine what foods may lead to health and longevity for the rest of us.

Since this work on the Blue Zones was first reported, scientists have been digging into the habits of these different populations and sharing their findings. I am going to share just a few of these research studies with you, because they give us a fascinating glimpse into the way long-living people enjoy foods that some of us may currently be afraid to eat based on the confusing messages we have heard over recent years. (Are these long-lived populations following a low-fat plan? Low carb? Ketogenic? No, no, and no.)

(Note: I know that you just read a whole chapter about how you should be cautious when someone cites scientific research, and this is the reason that I am including links to any scientific studies I mention. Remember: always go to the source and draw your own conclusions.)

Now, let's take a virtual field trip and travel the world to see what we can learn from these five distinct populations. First stop: Ikaria, Greece.

Ikaria is a Greek island located in the Mediterranean Sea. Scientists studied 1420 people (and then focused specifically on 89 men and 98 women over the age of 80) to determine what we might learn from them and how they live their lives. This became known as "The Ikaria Study." Here is a link to some of their results, which were published in 2011:

Scientists found that Ikaria had a higher percentage of the population over the age of 90 than was typical in other European counties. So: what do we know about how they eat?

If you go directly to that study, you can read a summary of the Ikarian "Lifestyle Characteristics." Particularly, take a look at Table 2. Within that table, you can see all sorts of interesting things about how these long-living Ikarians live, eat, and drink.

Their diets are Mediterranean in nature, and that means that they use a lot of olive oil in food preparation. They also favor fruits, vegetables, and salads as mainstays of their daily consumption. They eat potatoes several times per week. They include grains, legumes (such as beans), and fish. They also eat meat, and sweets, but not on a day-to-day basis.

What do they drink? Every day, they consume an average of 5 fl. oz. (150 mL) of alcohol, 10 fl. oz. (315 mL) of coffee, and about 3.5 fl. oz. (103 mL) of tea.

Finally, it's important to note that they actually don't eat much by American standards. The men that they studied report that they eat an average of 1,425 calories per day (+/- 532), and the women report eating an average of 1,087 calories per day (+/- 460). As a comparison, we can see what Americans were eating during that same 2009-2010 time-period. Based on information reported in the National Health and Nutrition Examination Study (NHANES), American men in the 70+ age group claimed to be eating an average of 1,907 calories per day, while the women in that same age group claimed to be eating an average of 1,535 calories per day. This information can be found here:

As you can see, Americans are eating a lot more food than the long-living Ikarians: about 500 more calories per day when we compare those above the age of 70. (As a side note, within this NHANES data, we can see that American men in the 20-29 age range were eating an average of 2,626 calories per day, while women in the 20-29 age range were eating an average of 1,949 calories per day. That is a lot more than both the older Americans and the Ikarians.)

Overall, after looking closely at the Ikarian Study, we can see that they eat a high proportion of plant-based foods, and they include both starches and grains, two foods that many Americans are hesitant to eat, based on the "carbs are bad" message. They enjoy coffee, tea, and alcohol, and they eat a lot less food than a typical Westerner.

After visiting Ikaria, we can travel westward across the Mediterranean Sea to the Italian island of Sardinia. This is where we will find the second Blue Zone, high in the mountains of this island.

Sardinia is in another part of the Mediterranean Sea than Ikaria, but they share many similarities. An article published in 2015 highlights what it is like to live in Sardinia:

Unfortunately, that is a link to the abstract only; I have read the actual article, though you will only be able to access the summary through that link.

So, what do they eat? According to the study, they traditionally eat a lot of grains, legumes, potatoes, and dairy products. They include plenty of fresh vegetables, some fruits, herbs, and nuts. It's notable that the amount of carbohydrate in their diet is surprisingly high. As with the

Ikarians, the long-living Sardinians don't eat a great deal of meat. Both the Ikarians and the Sardinians eat what could be categorized as a Mediterranean diet, high in plant-based foods. Olive oil and wine are staples.

Next, let's leave the Mediterranean and travel to Okinawa, Japan, and see what we can learn about longevity from this population in another of Buettner's Blue Zones. Interestingly, Okinawa is also located on an island, but this time, in the Pacific.

How is the Okinawan diet different from that of the Ikarians and the Sardinians? We can find the answers in a study called *Healthy Aging Diets Other than the Mediterranean: A Focus on the Okinawan Diet:*

https://www.ncbi.nlm.nih.gov/pmc/articles/PMC5403516/

When we read that study, we can see that the traditional Okinawan diet is what we call "nutrient dense." That means that on a calorie-by-calorie basis, the foods they eat are packed full of vitamins, minerals, and phytonutrients.

In the section of the paper called "'Haute cuisine' Okinawan style," we can find an image (Figure 1) showing a traditional Okinawan "food pyramid" of sorts. Traditionally, the Okinawans rely on vegetables and fruits as the mainstays of their diet, with sweet potatoes as a major staple. They also eat plenty of legumes (particularly soy) and grains (including rice), with a smaller proportion of their foods coming from fish and lean meats. They drink tea and a moderate amount of alcohol each day.

It's interesting to note that there is one other hypothesis about why the Okinawans may live so long, and that ties into their philosophy known as "Hara hachi bu." That phrase is attributed to Confucius, and means to eat until 80% full. As with the Ikarians, the Okinawans eat fewer overall calories than is typical in most Western populations. The scientific term for this is "calorie restriction," and this practice has been linked to longevity in many types of animals that have been studied. While the Okinawans, like the Ikarians, don't count calories, they also make sure not to overeat, as their "Hara hachi bu" philosophy reminds them.

As we leave Okinawa, the next stop on our trip around the world is Costa Rica. Costa Rica is not an island, but is located in Central America, with the Caribbean Sea to the east and the Pacific Ocean to the west.

How healthy are the long-living Costa Ricans? A 2008 study focused on the region's "nonagenarians," who are people living into their 90s and beyond. The study is called *The Exceptionally High Life Expectancy of Costa Rican Nonagenarians*, and the full study can be found here:

https://www.ncbi.nlm.nih.gov/pmc/articles/PMC2831395/

Besides enjoying a long life, according to that study, Costa Ricans have a 20% lower death rate from cardiovascular disease than Americans. Costa Ricans also have overall lower level of obesity and diabetes, and a smaller waist circumference.

Of course, we are interested in what they are eating. When we research to find their traditional diet, we find that as with the Okinawans, the Costa Ricans eat a lot of carbohydrates. Rice, beans, and corn are mainstays of their diet. They also eat plenty of vegetables and fruits, include dairy, and eat little meat. They rely on bananas and yams (yams are a root vegetable, and aren't the same thing as a sweet potato, even though we often use the terms interchangeably for some reason).

As we leave Costa Rica, the final stop on our tour of the Blue Zones takes us to the United States, of all places. Loma Linda, California is located east of Los Angeles, and is home to a large population of Adventists.

Seventh-day Adventists are a religious group with a strong belief in following what they consider to be Biblical food guidelines. The Adventists have been studied in great detail through the Adventist Health Studies (AHS and AHS-2), and the Loma Linda University Medical Center has a website devoted to their research:

http://publichealth.llu.edu/adventist-health-studies/findings/findings-ahs-2

According to their website, they have tracked thousands of Adventists over the years. Not all of the participants are from Loma Linda, though the research is being conducted there. This is because about a third of the population of Loma Linda itself is made up of Adventists.

Overall, Adventists typically eat a predominately plant-based diet with a small amount of dairy and meat. When divided into subgroups, some are vegetarian and include dairy/eggs (38%), some are vegan (8%), and another 6% do eat meat or fish infrequently. Almost half (48%) are non-vegetarian, meaning they eat animal products (red meat, poultry, fish, dairy, and eggs) more than once per week.

In their second longitudinal study (AHS-2), researchers compared the overall health outcomes of the Adventists who eat vegetarian diets to those who have an increased meat consumption. Results can be found here:

https://www.ncbi.nlm.nih.gov/pmc/articles/PMC4144107/

According to that study, the Adventists who follow the vegetarian dietary pattern had improved health outcomes related to BMI, diabetes, metabolic syndrome, hypertension, and overall mortality. It seems that the more vegetables and fruits they eat, the healthier they are, which is an important take away from this study.

We have now traveled to five different areas of the world to visit the longest-living people on earth: Ikaria, Greece; Sardinia, Italy; Okinawa, Japan; Costa Rica; and Loma Linda, California, in the United States. Even though we traveled virtually today, wouldn't it be an amazing trip to take one day? I would love to travel to each of these Blue Zones and have the chance to visit with the people in each region, sampling their regional dishes.

Now it's time to ask ourselves: are there any commonalities among these populations when it comes to what they eat?

The answer, of course, is yes. And it's striking. Every one of these populations, recognized for exceptional health and longevity, predominately eats a wide variety of foods from plants. This includes both grains and starchy vegetables such as potatoes, sweet potatoes, and yams. All of these populations eat dairy products. While they all eat meat, it is not the main focus of their diets. Most have moderate alcohol intake, and we also know that both the Ikarians and the Okinawans eat a lower volume of food (based on caloric intake) than those of us on a more typical Western diet.

One other thing that these populations have in common: they are all eating real food. This is important to understand. They aren't eating food-like products from a box or a pouch. They prepare foods in traditional ways. They celebrate throughout their lives with food, and they *Feast Without Fear*.

What can we take from these studies about the people in the Blue Zones? Think about it this way. Every diet book I've ever read is full of theory about how specific and individual foods and macronutrients "work" in the body. But, when we read about the longest living people in the world from the Blue Zones, this isn't theory based on results taken out of a lab. This isn't a scientist's idea of the "ideal human diet" based on mouse studies or a study of 10 people that was conducted over a 14-day period. No, this is about real people who have lived longer than most other people from around the world. We can see that their similar diets appear to be strongly correlated to positive health outcomes and longevity. I believe that they have a lot to teach us.

Now that we have explored the Blue Zones, we need to answer another question. Are there any other populations that prefer to eat the same types of foods as the long-living people from the Blue Zones? Actually, yes...and to find this population, we are going to have to travel deep inside of you...into your gut microbiome.

Chapter 6

Your amazing gut microbiome

Good news! Even though we just took a virtual field trip around the world to the Blue Zones, we are not going to take a field trip into your intestines, where your gut microbiome is located. You're welcome.

After all, deep inside your gut microbiome is probably not a very pleasant place to be...unless you are one of the trillions of bacterial cells residing there. Most of us don't spend a lot of time thinking about our gut region, but what goes on in this entirely unsexy part of your body is much more important than many people realize. How many bacteria live there? According to one estimate I read, if you took all of your gut bacteria and lined them up, one by one, the line would stretch from the earth to the moon. This population includes hundreds of different species, and it varies dramatically from person to person. Your specific gut microbiome is as unique as your fingerprint.

Based on everything I've been reading about the importance of the gut as it relates to our overall health, I don't think that it's a stretch to say that if your gut microbiome is unhealthy, then YOU are unhealthy. In fact, if your gut is unhealthy, you are more likely to be overweight, and you are also likely to have a hard time losing weight, no matter how hard you try.

I remember first hearing about the link between your gut microbiome and your weight years ago, when I was still overweight myself. I can't remember how I first heard about it, but the story sticks in my head.

According to what I remember, whatever article I read that day described how scientists took samples of the gut bacteria from obese mice and transplanted these samples into lean mice. This is known as a fecal transplant. With NO change in diet, the lean mice became obese themselves.

What?!?!?

Prior to that moment, I believed that losing weight was completely in our conscious control. I believed that if we had enough willpower and followed the right type of diet, we could and would lose weight. Isn't that what we all have been told? "Eat less, move more." If that isn't working, then it's because you are lazy, or you are a glutton, or, even worse, you are a lazy glutton. Suddenly, though, I had a new paradigm to consider. Was there something "wrong" with my gut microbiome that made it so hard for me to lose weight? Was it possible that it wasn't my fault, after all?

The problem was that even after reading about those mice, I still didn't know what to do about it. I remember going down to the health food store and wandering around the probiotic section. I knew that probiotics were supposed to improve gut health, but I had no idea where to begin, or which type to try. I bought some really expensive probiotics and started taking them. As with most things, I soon lost interest when I couldn't perceive any outward (or inward) changes. I mentally filed away the mouse study, hoping that one day we would know more about how to change our own gut microbiomes.

Well, that day is fast approaching, and it is completely thrilling.

Over the past decade or so, scientists have made some amazing discoveries about what actually lives in our gut. As new technologies have been developed, researchers are able to use genomic sequencing to identify the various bacterial species living deep within us. They are finding incredible correlations between specific species living in our gut and our overall health.

The story about fecal transplants in mice remained buried in my memory, until I heard another amazing story about the effect of the gut microbiome on weight. In 2015, scientists reported a case study about weight gain after a fecal transplant, this time in humans. Here is a link to the case study:

https://www.ncbi.nlm.nih.gov/pmc/articles/PMC4438885/

According to physicians, a woman received a fecal transplant as a treatment for an infection called *Clostridium difficile*. The official term for this procedure is a "Fecal Microbiota Transplant," or FMT. While it seems cringe-worthy, doctors take a sample from a stool donor and transfer it into the patient. The woman in this specific case selected her 16-year-old daughter as the donor. At the time of the FMT, the woman weighed 136 pounds, and her daughter weighed about 140 pounds.

Here's where the story gets interesting. 16 months later, at a follow up appointment, the woman had gained 34 pounds and was now classified as obese, with a BMI of 33. Prior to that, she never had any trouble with her weight. Suddenly, though, as hard as she tried, she was unable to lose weight, and kept steadily gaining. 36 months later, her weight was up even higher, leaving her with a BMI of 34.5. The odd part of the story is that the daughter also began to gain weight after the FMT, and ended up reaching 170 pounds herself.

Scientists hypothesized that since neither was obese prior to the FMT, either the procedure somehow triggered changes that led both women to gain weight, or prior to the transplant the daughter had an unhealthy gut microbiome that hadn't yet begun to affect her weight, and this only came to light after the procedure. As a result of this case, this specific physician's group created a policy to only use non-obese donors for any future FMTs. The funniest part of this whole case study is in the last paragraph of the paper, where the author discusses the use of "professional" stool donors for future procedures. Can you imagine that conversation at a cocktail party?

"So, Claude. What do you do for a living?"

"I'm a professional stool donor."

Claude would probably have trouble finding dates.

All jokes aside, the idea that we may be at the mercy of what resides in our gut is both fascinating and somewhat liberating, because if we can figure out how to correct imbalances in our gut, we should be able to affect our own health in many ways.

For an introduction into this fascinating world, I highly recommend that you read a comprehensive review article that appeared in "Integrative Medicine." This article is called *Part 1: The Human Gut Microbiome in Health and Disease.* Here is a link to the article, which you can read in its entirety:

https://www.ncbi.nlm.nih.gov/pmc/articles/PMC4566439/pdf/17-22.pdf

As we read about a healthy gut in this article, we learn that among the many types of bacteria present, there are 2 main phyla, or categories: Bacteroidetes and Firmicutes. The ratio of these 2 different types of bacteria seems to be different in the gut of lean creatures when compared to obese creatures, and obese mice (and humans) tend to have a higher proportion of Firmicutes, while lean mice (and humans) tend to have more Bacteroidetes. Yes, much of the research continues to be done using mice, as in the first study I remember hearing about, but we find many similarities as we move into human studies.

According to what we are learning, our gut microbiome affects both our metabolism and our immune system. In addition, scientists have discovered something called the gut-brain axis that shows that our gut is somewhat of a "second brain." Apparently, there is constant 2-way communication between our gut and our brain, and our behavior can even be affected by what resides in our gut. This gives a new meaning to the phrase "gut instinct", doesn't it?

In fact, scientists are finding that our gut microbiomes actually seem to somehow influence what foods we crave. An unhealthy gut microbiome has been linked to an increased preference for highly processed foods, and a more diverse and healthy gut microbiome appears to direct us to eat "healthier" foods. That's pretty remarkable, and it explains a lot.

So, how do our gut microbiomes end up in the states they are in currently, as either healthy or unhealthy? As it turns out, it's literally taken our whole lives to build whatever gut microbiome we currently have in place.

Let's go all the way back to the beginning. At the moment of our birth, microbial colonization begins. Researchers are finding that our method of birth actually has impact upon our microbiome: babies who are born vaginally have a more diverse population than those who are born by C-section. Throughout the first year of life, the microbiome continues to develop, and depends on many factors: whether you are breast or bottle fed, whether you need antibiotics, and when you begin solid food. Expect to hear more about this in coming years, because the more we learn about the microbiome, the more we realize that we can make a difference in our children's lives based on decisions we make starting at day one. In fact, just the other day, I saw a book targeted to pregnant women, all about developing your baby's gut microbiome. (One thing to note: it is at this point that some women begin to have guilt over having C-sections or bottle feeding their babies. STOP THIS GUILT, mothers, and understand that some factors are out of our control. If you had a C-section or bottle fed your baby, I am sure you did what you needed to do at that moment to keep your baby alive, which makes you a very good mother.)

Throughout our lives, our gut microbiomes continue to develop in response to what's around us and what we eat. It turns out that what we eat is very important in developing a healthy gut microbiome. What are the very worst things we can eat? You're probably not surprised to find that it's the modern-day Western diet, high in overly-processed and refined foods. Preservatives. Artificial sweeteners. Chemicals. All of these are implicated in an unhealthy gut microbiome. Oops. Apparently, it is our fault, after all. The unhealthy foods we chose to eat over the years weren't just "empty calories" as we were led to believe. No, it's much worse than that. These food choices were actually encouraging the growth of unhealthy bacterial species in our gut, at the expense of the beneficial ones.

When we feed our bodies foods that are both devoid of nutrients and highly processed, we end up with a microbiome that is out of balance. The result is inflammation, metabolic syndrome, and disease. Yes, all of these conditions can be linked back to an unhealthy gut. Here is an article that explains this further. It is called *Impact of the Gut Microbiota on Inflammation, Obesity, and Metabolic Disease*, and it can be found at this link:

https://genomemedicine.biomedcentral.com/track/pdf/10.1186/s13073-016-0303-2?site=genomemedicine.biomedcentral.com

So, we see that when our gut is out of balance, we end up with inflammation, metabolic disorders, excess fat accumulation, and insulin resistance. Now we can understand one reason why the Western diet is especially good at promoting obesity: it is specifically related to establishment of an unhealthy gut profile.

Here is something else that may absolutely shock you. When you have an unhealthy gut microbiome, your body is better at taking the energy from your food and storing it as fat. Yep, you read that correctly. You store MORE FAT from LESS FOOD than someone with a healthy gut microbiome.

If you always felt like you gained weight eating less food than the people around you, you were probably right. This is another reason why the calorie-model of weight loss fails. If you are able to extract more energy from your food, thanks to your gut microbiome, the calorie formulas aren't going to work very well for you. After "failing" at another calorie-restricted diet, it is as this point when many overweight people are accused of lying about what they are eating. Based on the calories in/calories out model, they should clearly be losing weight. But because of what is happening in their gut, they have different results.

Here is an example of that principle in action. Scientists have found that a specific type of "germ-free" mice typically eat 29% more calories than normal mice, yet they have 40% less body fat. These germ-free mice are also protected against insulin resistance. However, when a FMT is performed, transplanting microbes from normal mice, these germ-free mice see a 57% increase in body fat and a dramatic increase in insulin resistance, even when their diets are not changed at all.

According to this particular research, scientists have found that there are several ways that the gut microbiome affects energy balance and contributes to obesity. When we have the gut microbiome profiles that are correlated to obesity, we find that:
- More calories are extracted from the diet, meaning that more of the energy from our food is available to be stored as fat. This is known as "increased energy harvest."

- Our bodies become better at creating new fat deposits. This is known as "up-regulation of lipogenesis."
- Our bodies experience certain changes that make it more difficult to burn fat for fuel. One effect is that ketogenesis is downregulated (so it's harder to get into ketosis).

After learning all of this, we see that it is incredibly important to make choices that lead to the right kind of gut microbiome. I have good news for you! We can influence our guts positively in two ways: through fasting and by making certain food choices.

It's true! Fasting has been linked to beneficial changes in our gut microbiomes. One fascinating study was conducted in 2014, and results were reported in an article called *Increased Gut Microbiota Diversity and Abundance of Faecalibacterium Prausnitzii and Akkermansia After Fasting: A Pilot Study.* Here is a link to the study:

https://www.ncbi.nlm.nih.gov/pmc/articles/PMC4452615/pdf/508_2015_Article_755.pdf

In this study, scientists worked with thirteen overweight people to see what would happen to their gut microbiomes when they put them on a fasting regimen followed by probiotic supplementation. (Okay, 13 people is a very small sample size. Keep that in mind. Even so, the research is interesting.) They spent one week on the fasting protocol, and then spent six weeks ingesting a specific probiotic formula. Fecal samples were taken before the study began, during the fasting portion of the protocol, and after the probiotic treatment.

The scientists found that as a result of the fasting protocol and subsequent probiotic treatment, there was an increase in microbial diversity, with a specific increase in *Akkermansia* and *Bifidobacteria*. Both of those species are associated with a lean and healthy gut profile. *Akkermansia* is specifically associated with fasting, as it is a species that lives on the mucus in your gut lining. This is just another reason to feel good about your decision to adopt an intermittent fasting lifestyle!

So: what do our gut microbiomes like to eat? Besides *Akkermansia*, who thrive when we are fasting, there are other species who need specific foods that they can only get from what we send down to them. When we feed the good guys in our guts, they are able to crowd out the bad guys over time. The types of foods that best feed our good guys can be called "prebiotics." Note that this is not a typo. Prebiotics differ from probiotics.

Prebiotics are foods, primarily composed of oligosaccharides or short-chain polysaccharides. One famous prebiotic fiber is inulin, which you may have heard of. While we can supplement our prebiotic intake with certain prebiotic supplements, the most powerful way to feed our gut bacteria is to consume prebiotic foods.

As I already mentioned, a Western diet of highly processed and nutrient-deficient foods is terrible for our gut microbiome. To find out how we should (and shouldn't) be feeding our microbiome, we can look to a paper called *Starving our Microbial Self: The Deleterious Consequences of a Diet Deficient in Microbiota-Accessible Carbohydrates.* Here is a link to this paper:

http://ac.els-cdn.com/S1550413114003118/1-s2.0-S1550413114003118-main.pdf?_tid=2d5412ec-627f-11e7-8e8a-00000aacb361&acdnat=1499368582_c416582e5d4b852458f9de95206a6147

The authors of this paper suggest that we need to ensure a diet high in what they call "microbiota-accessible carbohydrates," or MACs, in order to have a healthy gut microbiome. MACs are specific carbohydrates that are broken down in the gut by our bacterial good guys. Think about foods high in dietary fiber. Your grandmother was right: we need to eat more fiber.

Here's something interesting, though. The carbohydrates that best feed MY gut microbiome might be different from the carbohydrates that best feed YOUR gut microbiome. Our genes play a role in this to a degree, as does the specific composition of our unique gut microbiomes.

Overall, though, we know that certain prebiotic foods tend to feed our gut microbiomes well. These include a wide variety of vegetables, fruits, and whole grains. The good news is that if you eat a wide variety of these foods, you are on the right track: diversity is key, and we want to have a lot of variety from day to day. Foods high in something called "resistant starch" are also great for our gut microbiomes. We find resistant starch in foods such as beans, grains, and seeds.

We also find high levels of resistant starch in certain foods that have been cooked and then cooled, such as rice, pasta, or potatoes. What changes when we cook and then cool these starches? Think about a baked potato straight out of the oven for a minute. It's fluffy and soft. Now, think about what happens to the texture of that potato if you let it completely cool. You'll never be able to get the fluffy texture back. The potato underwent structural changes as a result of the cooking and cooling process, and for that reason, it is less digestible within our bodies. It is, however, now a great source of resistant starch, and it will make it to our gut, where it will feed our good gut bacteria. In addition to feeding the good guys, these cooked and then cooled resistant starches lead to a smaller increase in both blood glucose levels and insulin after eating them, as compared to when they were first cooked. Time to bring out the cold potato salad recipes!

Besides feeding our gut microbiomes a wide variety of prebiotic foods, we can also increase probiotic foods to promote gut health. We all have heard of yogurt, with its probiotic properties. Fermented foods, such as sauerkraut, kefir, and kimchi, are also great sources of probiotics.

I'm sure by now you are as fascinated as I am by the possibilities the lie within our gut microbiomes. Starting today, you can work to add prebiotic and probiotic foods into your diet. The more variety you include, the better for your diverse gut microbiome. You can also feel good about incorporating an intermittent fasting regimen. In addition, every time you choose a high quality real food over a highly processed food, you can be sure you are making a great choice for your body. Now you understand why it matters so much.

But, what if you think that your gut microbiome is probably in terrible shape? What if you have a suspicion that you are one of those people that needs to make substantial changes in your microbiome? If you have metabolic issues, increased inflammation, and other health conditions, you probably do need to take more drastic steps to change your gut microbiome.

I am not going to tell you how to heal your gut microbiome, because that is beyond the scope of this particular book. Remember, I am a teacher and not a doctor. Hopefully, I have taught you how important a healthy gut microbiome is to your overall health, but you need to consult with physicians (or read their books) to learn how to heal your own microbiome. I do have some recommended reading for you, however. There are already several great books about the gut microbiome, and I'm sure there are more in the works, as we continue to recognize the importance of the gut microbiome to our overall health and wellness.

If you just want to read more about the gut microbiome, I highly recommend *The Diet Myth*, by Tim Spector. He is the lead scientist with the British Gut Project, and his book is fascinating. The most important takeaway from his book, in my opinion, has to do with avoiding any restrictive diet that limits the variety of foods that we eat. When we follow a restrictive diet, such as one that eliminates an entire group of macronutrients (as in a program that restricts carbohydrates, and particularly the microbiota-accessible carbs), this leads to a further reduction of diversity in our gut. As we have seen, this is NOT a good thing, and while this type of restrictive diet may seem to correct problems in the short-term, the long-term impact may be detrimental to our gut microbiome.

My favorite parts of *The Diet Myth* are Tim Spector's personal stories, which are sprinkled throughout the book. He talks candidly about what he eats, and why. When a scientist who researches the gut microbiome tells me what he himself is eating, I make sure to pay attention. He suggests eating a wide variety of foods, heavily skewed towards vegetables, fruits, beans, nuts, and olive oil. He endorses traditional cheeses, and high-quality yogurts (but not the high sugar/low fat variety.) He also cautions against overly processed foods, and recommends eating less meat overall.

Another book that just came out in mid-2017 is *The Clever Guts Diet*, written by Dr. Michael Mosely. (This is the title of the British version; I believe the American version will have a slightly different title.) This book is a great summary of what scientists have learned about the gut microbiome, and he goes well beyond what I have shared with you in this chapter. Dr. Mosely also has a 2-stage plan for healing your gut microbiome that you may find to be of value.

If you are interested, you can actually have your microbiome analyzed to find out what you are working with. Both The British Gut Project and The American Gut Project have programs that allow you to send in a specimen for them to analyze. I am waiting for my results now, as a matter of fact. I am sure you aren't surprised to hear that I am participating in this type of analysis. Reading their report should be as exciting as Christmas morning, now that I understand how important our gut microbiome is. When I mailed off my "sample" I was really glad that the lady at the post office didn't ask me what was in the package. Awkward.

If you believe your gut problems go beyond what you may be able to correct through reading a book and making simple dietary changes, you may need to consult a physician who works with the gut. If you suspect that you have sensitivities to grains, dairy, etc., there are things that you and a doctor can do to point you in the direction of healing. Your overall goal would be to heal any underlying issues so you can reintroduce foods that you would like to eat.

Also, one thing I want to mention. If you are working on gut health at home, it's important to understand that you don't want to make too many changes at once. If you completely change your diet by adding in a lot more fiber than you are used to, coupled with a lot of probiotic foods, it may feel like World War III is being fought inside of you. You may feel a lot worse than you did before you started, and you'll be cursing the day that you ever took any of my advice. So, start slow. Make one change at a time. You'll be glad you did.

Now that we understand how important it is to feed our gut microbiomes well, let's see if we can connect this information to what we read in the chapter about the Blue Zones.

Chapter 7

Connecting the dots: Blue Zones to microbiomes

When I first read about the Blue Zones a few years ago, I thought it was interesting, and I mentally filed it away for future reference. The same is true for what I read about the gut microbiome and how it was important for overall health. I read some things about it, and mentally filed it away, as well.

When I decided to write this book, and dig through everything science could tell us, I found my way back to both the Blue Zones and the gut microbiome. As I filtered through all of the dietary noise about what we "should" be eating, I took a fresh look at what the longest living people in the world are eating, and at what foods seem to encourage the kind of microbial diversity that is correlated to vibrant health.

Talk about an a-ha moment.

When I put the two sets of dietary recommendations side by side, the patterns that emerged literally blew me away.

In case you haven't already figured it out: the foods that the people in the Blue Zones eat are primarily the same types of foods that our gut microbiomes thrive upon. Let that sink in for a moment. The people who live the longest in the world eat the same types of foods that encourage the type of diversity we want in our gut microbiomes.

Wow.

We can also take something else away from this realization. In contrast to the whole foods that the long-lived Blue Zones residents eat, the types of foods that we are eating as a part of a typical Western diet, which are making us sicker and sicker, are the exact foods that are linked to decreased diversity in our gut microbiomes.

When we eat like those who live in the Blue Zones, we are eating in a way that encourages diversity in our gut. Some of these foods, such as whole grains, may be a surprise to some, because we have it so ingrained in our diet-psyche that "carbs are bad." In fact, when you ask people why they are overweight, many of them might say, "too many carbs." Yet, our gut microbiomes thrive on many types of carbs, and if we restrict these types of carbs long term, we are left with less microbial diversity. We now know that decreased microbial diversity isn't good for us. The long-living residents of the Blue Zones actually thrive on what would be described by many as high-carb diets. Clearly, it's not as simple as "carbs are bad," as many of us have been led to believe.

Besides the evidence from the Blue Zones and the research being conducted on our gut microbiomes, can we find any other compelling scientific evidence in support of this type of eating pattern, which is high in carbohydrates from plant sources? The answer is yes. Let's take a look at some of the latest studies to see what science is teaching us about the relationship between what we eat and specific health outcomes, such as heart disease, metabolic syndrome, and diabetes.

Chapter 8

The Mediterranean diet: Research

When we look for high–quality scientific research, we want to see a large sample size, and we also want to see that the study was conducted over a long period of time. In addition, we hope that the scientists were able to control as many variables as possible, considering that they are dealing with people, who are most definitely not all the same and clearly uncontrollable on many occasions. (As a teacher, I know this.) Fortunately, the PREDIMED trial meets many of these criteria fairly well.

PREDIMED stands for "Prevencion con Dieta Mediterranea," which is Spanish for "I am not sure exactly because I don't speak Spanish, but I know they were studying the effects of a Mediterranean diet on various health outcomes." This study, which began in 2003 and lasted until 2010, investigated the relationship between a Mediterranean diet and various health outcomes. Fortunately for me, their results have all been published in English.

Before we get into specifics, let's define what we mean by a "Mediterranean diet." This type of eating pattern is generally high in fruits and vegetables, and also includes plenty of legumes (beans), fish, whole grains, nuts and seeds, and olive oil. You'll find a more moderate intake of dairy products and wine, with a lower overall consumption of certain foods, including red and processed meats and foods with a high sugar content.

To design and oversee this large-scale research study, scientists in Spain collaborated with others from around the world, including researchers from Columbia University, Harvard University, and Loma Linda University. They enrolled 7,447 participants between the ages of 55-80, all of whom were judged to be at "high risk" of cardiovascular disease (CVD) at the beginning of the study. This means that all of the participants in the study had three or more risk factors for CVD, including Type 2 diabetes, high blood pressure, smoking, poor cholesterol profiles, obesity, and/or a family history of CVD.

Participants were divided into three groups:
- A Mediterranean diet with supplemental extra virgin olive oil.
- A Mediterranean diet with supplemental tree nuts.
- A control diet, modeled after the current American Heart Association low-fat eating recommendations.

These three groups were then followed for about 5 years to assess the effect of these dietary patterns on their overall health, and specifically their cardiovascular outcomes. None of the participants were asked to limit calorie intake or increase exercise.

If you want to watch a short video (about 15 minutes) as an introduction to their study methods, here is a link to one:

https://youtu.be/AEsVDmPnGdw

The video is called "Presentation of the Final Results [PREDIMED]", and it explains how the participants were selected and placed into groups so that each group was as similar as possible to the other groups.

Of course, as I mentioned before in a previous chapter, one limitation to this type of research is that it can be difficult to ascertain whether participants in a study followed the prescribed dietary recommendations, so it's important to know that the researchers conducted interviews frequently with the participants to see if they were following the guidelines outlined in the plans. To measure adherence, participants met with dieticians who determined if they were, indeed, eating according to recommendations. A questionnaire was used to rate participants' levels of compliance. It is possible that participants weren't honest with the researchers about what they were eating? Sure.

At the conclusion of the study in 2013, initial results were published, in a paper called *Primary Prevention of Cardiovascular Disease with a Mediterranean Diet*, which is available at this link:

http://www.unav.edu/departamento/preventiva/fil es/file/predimed/NEJM_PREDIMED_printed.pdf

At that link, you can find more details about how the study was conducted. Remember: it's always best to look at something for yourself in order to draw conclusions about results, rather than just take my word for it.

The most exciting information in this paper is found in the discussion section. According to the authors, they found that the two Mediterranean diet groups had a 30% risk-reduction for cardiovascular events during the study, when compared to the control diet group. The two Mediterranean diet groups also had a lowered risk of stroke. Remember that the participants were selected because they were at a high risk for cardiovascular disease: they all had 3 or more risk factors, and they were all between the ages of 55-80. To substantially lower the risk for cardiovascular events within this population is impressive, since they were all considered to be high-risk at the beginning of the study. These results were all due to dietary interventions alone, and not based on medications.

To learn more about the PREDIMED trial specifically, all of their published research is available to you at their website:

http://www.predimed.es/publications.html

Through this link, you have access to paper after paper showing the amazing benefits attributed to the Mediterranean diet. I encourage you to dig into these studies to see what you can learn.

The PREDIMED study is not the only one to investigate the benefits of a Mediterranean diet. In fact, scientists have been investigating the effectiveness of a Mediterranean diet for years. While PREDIMED is the most ambitious study undertaken thus far, other studies also support this particular dietary pattern. Some of the key research from these studies has been summarized in a paper called *Protective Effects of the Mediterranean Diet on Type 2 Diabetes and Metabolic Syndrome*, which is available here:

https://www.ncbi.nlm.nih.gov/pmc/articles/PMC4807638/

This paper does an excellent job discussing many of the various studies and what was found. I highly encourage you to read it.

In one meta-analysis of studies related to the Mediterranean diet, researchers found 20 studies with dietary interventions that lasted for more than 6 months. Overall, they found that the Mediterranean dietary pattern showed greater improvement in both glycemic control and insulin sensitivity when compared to other diets. Based on what we know about insulin and weight management, we understand that insulin sensitivity is associated with better health outcomes long-term.

Besides clinical trials, some of the Mediterranean diet studies were epidemiologic in nature, meaning that the study attempted to link specific health results to certain factors within the participants' lifestyles. While these types of studies do have some limitations, and may not give us as much information as well done clinical trials, common results were discovered among these studies:

- All of the studies demonstrated a protective role of the Mediterranean diet against Type 2 diabetes. Among the studies reported, the risk reduction ranged from 12%-83%.
- In a meta-analysis of all studies reported from 2007-2014, a higher adherence to a Mediterranean diet pattern was associated with a 19% lower diabetes risk.
- One study following 2,563 Spanish participants for 6 years found that following a Mediterranean diet was associated with an 80% lower risk of Metabolic Syndrome.
- In another study, which followed 1,918 participants for 7 years, those who followed a Mediterranean dietary pattern had a 30% lower risk of Metabolic Syndrome when compared to those who were least compliant.

One specific study is interesting because it takes us back to the Blue Zone located in Loma Linda, California. Results of a study (using the Adventists that we learned about earlier) were reported in a paper called *Intake of Mediterranean Foods Associated with Positive Affect and Low Negative Affect*, which can be found here:

https://www.ncbi.nlm.nih.gov/pmc/articles/PMC3790574/pdf/nihms512849.pdf

By now, it shouldn't surprise you that results of this study indicated that the more fresh vegetables, fruits, olive oil, nuts, and legumes participants ate, the better their overall health outcomes.

So, you might ask: do we have sufficient evidence to point toward a Mediterranean dietary pattern as superior to other eating styles? A group of experts from France, Germany, Italy, Portugal, Spain, and Switzerland would say that the answer to that question is yes.

Recently, this team of experts (including cardiologists, endocrinologists, and internists) got together and examined all of the evidence related to dietary recommendations and health outcomes. Their 2017 report is called *Is There a Role for Lifestyle Changes in Cardiovascular Prevention? What, When, and How?* The full report in pdf format can be found here:

http://www.sciencedirect.com/science/article/pii/S156756881730020X

Their overall dietary recommendations can be seen throughout the paper. Based upon the most recent scientific understandings, this group of physicians felt strongly that the best dietary pattern includes plenty of fruits and vegetables, seeds, nuts, fish, whole grains, and olive oil. As you know, this is typical of what is found in a Mediterranean diet. Rather than think of specific foods found only in the Mediterranean region, however, the physicians felt that anyone could adapt these recommendations to include foods that are available to us locally that meet these criteria. That is: eat plenty of whatever fruits, vegetables, seeds, nuts, fish, and whole grains are available to you.

These experts also agreed that there is no evidence to support a low-fat diet, though they did recommend getting most of the fat in our diets from plant sources such as olive oil. (In a later chapter about genetic differences, we will see that some people need to worry more about saturated fat than others, based on individual differences.)

To read what some other experts have to say about the Mediterranean dietary pattern, including their recommendations of what to eat and how it has been shown to affect various health outcomes, you can read *Definitions and Potential Health Benefits of the Mediterranean Diet: Views from Experts Around the World:*

In this paper, 8 different experts share their thoughts. In addition, there is an image called the *Mediterranean Diet Pyramid* (Figure 5) that includes specific dietary guidelines for what a Mediterranean dietary pattern generally looks like.

While we know that there are limitations to be found with all scientific studies, the accumulation of evidence is pretty compelling. If you have been paying attention (and the teacher in me hopes that you have), you may have noticed that the types of foods associated with a healthy Mediterranean diet are similar to the foods eaten in the Blue Zones. These foods are also the ones that seem to feed our gut microbiomes the best.

Now, let's put all of this information together and see what foods we can confidently add to our diets so we can *Feast Without Fear*!

Chapter 9

Farewell to fear

After everything I have learned, the emerging picture seems pretty clear. The foods that the longest living people in the world feast upon are the same foods that feed our gut microbiomes well. These are also the same foods associated with positive health outcomes in study after study about the power of a Mediterranean-type diet. When we add these foods to our plates, we can *Feast Without Fear.*

Some of these foods may include items you believe that you should avoid if you're a long-term dieter. This is because when we focus on specific macronutrients, as many diet books do, we tend to fixate on whether a food is a "carb" or a "fat", and we then lump all carbs and fats into one category as either "good" or "bad." Actually, though, our bodies need all macronutrients. In fact, it can be said that the overall *quality* of the foods we choose is a lot more important than the ratio of the macronutrients found in these foods.

The long-living people in the Blue Zones don't count calories or restrict macronutrients. Participants in most of the studies related to the Mediterranean diet weren't counting calories or restricting macronutrients, either. The bacteria living in our gut thrive on a wide variety of foods, and the greater the diversity of what we send down to them, the healthier our gut microbiomes will be.

If you want to *Feast Without Fear,* you need to follow the lessons from all three of these sources: eat a wide variety of real foods.

It is important for us to realize: we should no longer fear "carbs" or "fats" or even "protein." Or grains. Or beans. Or dairy. Or meat. Don't fear any real foods that humans have been eating for generations. The key is "real foods."

Remember that a healthy gut microbiome prefers real foods to overly processed foods. These are the same types of foods that are linked to longevity in populations from around the world. These are also the types of foods linked to lowered risk of obesity, Type 2 diabetes, and cardiovascular risk in study after study on the benefits of the Mediterranean diet.

Does that mean that every person will be able to eat exactly the same way and get precisely the same results? No, and we will discuss that in the next chapter. We do have individual differences that make it impossible to have any one-size-fits-all meal plan.

Still, though, we can use these overall recommendations (from the Blue Zones, Mediterranean diets, and what feeds our gut microbiomes well) to develop a template of what foods work well for most people (see chapter 14!) Once we do that, we understand that we can and should include a wide variety of foods into our diets without fear.

When we *Feast Without Fear,* it's important to reframe our thinking. As an example, we should not be afraid of "carbs," but we should make sure to add in the right types of carbs. What does that look like? Think about real fruits and vegetables that are close to their natural state. Choose whole grains that have not been overly refined. Yes, there is a place in our lives for bread dipped in olive oil. We can enjoy a glass of wine with dinner.

Even with all of the evidence from the Blue Zones, the gut microbiome research, and the Mediterranean diet studies, one fact remains: we are all different genetically.

86

Do these differences affect what foods may or may not work well for us individually? Of course, the answer is yes.

Chapter 10

It's in your genes

As I mentioned in the gut microbiome chapter, our bodies are home to trillions of other living creatures that call us home. I also mentioned how certain gut profiles are associated with various disease states, so we understand that individual differences within our gut microbiomes will affect what foods work best for us.

It should come as no surprise to you that we have other differences that affect both what foods work well for us and how our bodies gain and lose weight, and you may have already figured out that I am talking about genetic differences.

Scientists are finding that genetic differences most definitely play a role in how our unique bodies respond to foods, and it's fascinating. I want to warn you: this may be the most science-y chapter in the whole book, so be prepared. This field is still emerging and also very complex, so I hope I don't do a terrible job explaining it to you (if you are a geneticist, feel free to cringe if I have oversimplified or gotten something slightly wrong within the chapter).

Ready to dig in?

What better way to examine genetic differences than to study identical twins, since they begin life with the same genetic profile. In one fascinating study called *The Response to Long-Term Overfeeding in Identical Twins*, researchers studied 12 pairs of male identical twins to see what would happen if they fed them more calories than they needed to maintain their body weights. The study is found here:

http://www.nejm.org/doi/pdf/10.1056/NEJM19900
5243222101

These 24 men were studied over a 120-day period, and they were housed in a special dorm while under 24-hour supervision. In the first two weeks, researchers allowed them to eat freely, and therefore determined their average caloric intake for weight maintenance.

After the first two weeks, each participant was fed a diet containing 1,000 more calories per day than their maintenance level (six days out of the week), with one day per week at their maintenance calorie level. This continued for a total of 84 days of overfeeding. Based on the calories in/calories out model of weight management, we would expect them all to gain the same amount of weight, right? After all, if "a calorie is a calorie," and every pound of weight gain comes from overeating by 3,500 calories, which is what most of us have been told, then feeding these men an extra 1,000 calories per day would lead to one pound of weight gain for every 3 ½ days of overfeeding. It's simple math, right? After "overeating" a total of 84,000 calories over the period of the study, each young man should have mathematically gained exactly 24 pounds. Is that what happened?

No.

In fact, Table 1 of that paper tells us that the average weight gain was actually 8.1 kg, which translates into about 18 pounds. Instead of gaining the predicted 24 pounds, based on the simple math of the calories in/calories out (CI/CO) model, the average gain was 6 pounds less than expected. Oops. Another nail in the coffin of the CI/CO model. None of these young men had bodies that worked like a calorie calculator, as we all should understand by now.

Here's where it becomes even more interesting. The actual amount of weight gained varied tremendously from person to person, with a low of 4.3 kg, or 9 ½ pounds, and a high of 13.3 kg, or about 29 pounds. Yep, that one poor guy gained about 5 MORE pounds than the CI/CO model would predict. Oops again. And that one lucky fellow gained about 14 fewer pounds than predicted. Also, some of the young men gained a higher proportion of fat to lean tissue than others, showing that their bodies didn't respond in the same way to the extra calories. Some of the young men had an increase in metabolic rate in response to the overfeeding, while others didn't.

Besides showing us once again that we can't count on the CI/CO model to predict weight gain precisely, we can learn something else from their results. They found that the identical twins had significant similarities in the amount of weight they gained, how much of it was fat vs. muscle, and where the fat was distributed. As a result of their findings, the authors concluded that genetic factors were most likely involved, and these genetic factors may determine whether individuals are more likely to gain excess fat or muscle mass after overfeeding. Of course, we know that the gut microbiome also plays a role in determining what our bodies do with the calories we eat, though this particular study was conducted in 1990, which was before scientists knew how to determine the identity of the specific strains of bacteria that live in our gut. Now we know that our gut profiles may ultimately be even more important than genetics, but even so, genetic differences still remain an important factor.

We are still learning about how our specific genes may influence our weight and health. In a paper called *Gene-diet Interaction and Weight Loss*, some of the research has been reviewed and summarized. This paper is available here:

https://www.ncbi.nlm.nih.gov/pmc/articles/PMC5330198/pdf/nihms846027.pdf

According to the authors, scientists are beginning to connect specific genetic factors to success of various diets. When individual genotypes are taken into account, specific dietary interventions have been shown to work differently from person to person. That's pretty exciting to understand, because it explains why a diet may have worked well for your friend but not at all for you.

In one 2-year study of about 800 participants called POUNDS LOST (short for "Preventing Overweight Using Novel Dietary Strategies"), researchers found that the macronutrient content of the various diets did not have an overall effect on weight loss when all of the participants were viewed as a whole. There was not one "best" macronutrient ratio for weight loss. However, when participants were analyzed based on specific genetic factors, a different picture emerged.

First, a little background information. When we look at our genetic profiles, we examine something called the "Single Nucleotide Polymorphisms," or SNPs (pronounced "snips.") These SNPs (which are identified by number) vary from person to person, and scientists are able to associate specific SNP profiles with certain outcomes. For each SNP, individuals can be categorized as a specific genotype. Don't get too hung up on the terminology, because it gets a bit overwhelming. Just remember this: each SNP has more than one genotype associated with it, and these genotypes are identified by letters.

Now, back to the study. When researchers conducting the POUNDS LOST study analyzed participants based on a specific SNP (numbered rs2943641), they found that certain genotypes had significant differences in response to diet composition. As an example, those with the CC genotype for that particular SNP lost less weight and had higher fasting insulin levels when they followed a higher carbohydrate diet. So, when you talk to your friend who had great success on a low carb plan, you can guess that your friend may be a CC genotype when it comes to SNP rs2943641.

Also in the POUNDS LOST trial, other genetic differences were found based on a different SNP: rs1558902. Participants with a TT genotype for that SNP lost more weight and had better results with a low protein diet, while those with the AA genotype had better results with a high protein diet. Results are reported in an article called *FTO Genotype and 2-Year Change in Body Composition and Fat Distribution in Response to Weight Loss Diets: The POUNDS LOST Trial.* A link to this paper is found here:

https://www.ncbi.nlm.nih.gov/pmc/articles/PMC3478519/pdf/3005.pdf

Based on that research, I'm pretty sure that if you read a diet book recommending a high-protein approach as the absolute path to weight loss success for all, I would bet that the author probably has the AA genotype, and the high-protein approach worked best for him. Does that mean it will work best for everyone? Of course not, since it most likely won't work well for those of us with the TT genotype.

Scientists are learning more and more about how our genes influence our health and our metabolisms, including our body weight. The good news is that you can have this type of testing done, and you actually may already have done it without realizing it.

Several companies now offer genetic testing where you provide a saliva sample through the mail and they send you a report about your ancestry and certain other characteristics. Both my husband and I had this done, because we were interested in discovering where our ancestors lived. We were both surprised at what we learned, which didn't match what our families believed to be true. We each found fascinating stuff within our ancestry reports.

However, the most interesting information is found deep within the raw genetic data, and you can find out a lot more about yourself than simply where your ancestors were from. The company I used for my initial analysis allows you to export your raw data from their platform, and you can then use third-party sites to analyze your data further. There is so much information available that it can actually be overwhelming.

I had a lot of fun looking at my raw data through one of these third-party sites. You can type in the SNP numbers that you are interested in and find your specific genotypes for each. SNP rs1558902? I'm a TT. That means that I should have better results with a low protein approach to weight loss, based on what I learned by studying the POUNDS LOST Trial. (Is it a coincidence that I feel better when I eat less meat? I don't think so.) SNP rs2943641? I'm a CT. I was actually hoping for CC, which was the group associated with better results on the high-carb plan (and I love carbs!) SNP rs1801282? I'm a CC for that one, which means I have a "normal fat metabolism." That sounds good to me!

If you aren't willing to brave the raw data on your own, you can still get a lot of information from the basic reports provided by the company. The company I used analyzes several basic areas and provides you with a summary of the results.

According to the company's report, based on my variants related to a gene called APOA2, I am an AG. This means I am likely to do equally well on a diet that is high or low in saturated fat. Other people (GG) are likely to gain more weight on a diet high in saturated fat. Your friends who did very well on the low-fat diets popular in the 1990s probably have the GG genotype. They tend to be healthier when they avoid saturated fat in their diets.

Another report of interest to me was the one analyzing my likelihood to be lactose intolerant. Based on my results, I have the AA genotype, meaning I am likely NOT lactose intolerant. Hooray for that, because I enjoy dairy products. Much of the world, however, has the GG variant, meaning that they probably don't do well with dairy. The diet books that encourage us to all avoid dairy are probably written by authors with the GG variant, as they are likely to feel better without dairy.

One last report that I found to be interesting was the "Genetic Weight" report. According to all of my genetic data, my genes predispose me to weigh about average. The report went on to tell me that my current weight is actually lower than my genetic result would predict by about 30 pounds. (Thank you, intermittent fasting. This is one time when I am happy to be below average!)

How does understanding our genetic differences help us to *Feast Without Fear*? Well, we can understand that our individual genetic differences most likely affect which foods work best for our unique genetic profiles, which helps us to take one more step away from the diet world. When we understand that we have unique genetic profiles, we know that any type of universal dietary advice about specific macronutrients, such as protein, carbohydrates, and fat, is useless. If I told a person with an TT genotype for SNP rs1558902 to eat more protein in order to lose weight, that would probably be the exact wrong advice. If I told a person with the CC genotype for rs2943641 to add more carbs in order to lose more weight, that would most likely be a terrible recommendation. And if I told a person with the GG variation for APOA2 to eat more saturated fat, it probably would be the complete wrong suggestion.

Now then. Even though I have just spent the first part of the chapter explaining that our genes play a role in determining what foods work best for each of us, I am going to share some of the most cutting-edge research being done in the field. Are you ready to have your mind blown yet again by science?

Thanks to groundbreaking work being done through the Human Genome Project, scientists are finding out that even though we are predisposed to certain outcomes based on our individual genes, very little is actually set in stone, the way we may have previously believed.

94

When you were in school, you probably studied dominant and recessive genes, and made those Punnett squares to figure out the probabilities of having offspring with specific characteristics. Remember those? You may have calculated your probability of having blue eyes based on your parents' eye colors, or figured out what color fur a rabbit could have, based on the parents' fur colors.

You may not know that there are actually very few gene variants that give us fixed characteristics, and instead, most gene variants simply predispose us to certain characteristics, diseases, or behaviors. So, earlier in the chapter when I discussed the study that related protein intake to weight loss, and I mentioned that someone with a TT variation is more likely to do well on a low protein diet, that doesn't mean that the results are set in stone. The same thing is true for most of our gene variants. These gene variants only tell us what might happen.

New findings in genetic research point to the importance of something called your *epigenome*. According to the National Institutes of Health (NIH), "*The epigenome comprises all of the chemical compounds that have been added to the entirety of one's DNA (genome) as a way to regulate the activity (expression) of all the genes within the genome. The chemical compounds of the epigenome are not part of the DNA sequence, but are on or attached to DNA.*"

Whew! That's pretty science-y. What does it mean?

Here is a link to the National Institutes of Health National Human Genome Research Institute's explanation of epigenetics:

https://www.genome.gov/27532724/epigenomics-fact-sheet/

Basically, what this means is that we have chemical compounds on or around our DNA that tell our genes what to do. These compounds direct what actually happens within our bodies, including how the genes are expressed.

Both lifestyle and environmental factors can cause changes within our epigenomes leading to changes in the way our cells use the instructions found within our actual DNA code.

This means that genes can be switched on and off, like a light switch. Our genes react to our experiences! Things are much less set in stone than we thought.

The reason I mention epigenetics and gene expression is because I don't want you to think that you can get a DNA report and blindly follow the dietary recommendations within it. For one thing, this science is in its infancy, and many of the studies are small. For another, we now realize that what's written in your DNA is far from a life sentence, but instead is simply a set of possibilities.

Yes, we can use the information about our genetic differences to understand that we have predispositions to certain outcomes, but overall, we still retain some control over these outcomes. If you are interested in learning more about how you can affect your gene expression in powerful ways, I highly recommend a book called *Super Genes: Unlock the Power of your DNA for Optimum Health and Well-Being*. It was written by Dr. Rudolph Tanzi (a professor of Neurology from Harvard) and Dr. Deepak Chopra (an MD who embraces alternative and integrative medicine). It's a fascinating read.

So: we now understand that we have genetic differences that may shape what foods are likely to work best for us, and also that our unique gut microbiomes cause each of us to have different results when it comes to specific foods. Scientists are now taking the research to a more personalized level, which I will share in the next chapter.

Chapter 11

The era of personalized nutrition

Are you ready to have your mind blown again? If you are near a computer, you need to take a few minutes to watch a YouTube video of a TedTalk given by Dr. Eran Segal called *What is the Best Diet for Humans?* You can search for it by title on YouTube, or you can access it at this link:

https://youtu.be/0z03xkwFbw4

The video is only 19 minutes long, but the information is incredible. You have probably heard about the glycemic index.   You may believe, as I once did, that our bodies all respond pretty much the same way to foods. When it comes to the glycemic index, we have been given certain numerical values for various foods, and most of us think that these numbers represent the glycemic response that we should all expect from eating these same foods. Well, research is showing that's not true.

Dr. Segal and his research group published some surprising results in 2015, in an article called *Personalized Nutrition by Prediction of Glycemic Response*, and it can be viewed here:

http://www.cell.com/cell/pdf/S0092-8674(15)01481-6.pdf

Dr. Segal and his team hypothesized that each person would respond differently to various foods, based on individual differences related to genetics and their gut microbiomes. (Sound familiar?) To determine which foods worked best for each person, they decided to use the "meal glucose response," which refers to the blood glucose changes that each participant experiences after eating. Based on what we know about how the body works, a high glucose response after a meal is associated with weight gain, and an overall pattern showing high glucose spikes after eating is a risk factor for many metabolic disorders, such as Type 2 diabetes.

The first step in their research was to find 800 healthy adults, and to equip them each with a glucose sensor. They were able to track the participants' blood glucose levels continually for a week. After eating, each participant logged meals using an app, and the researchers had data showing how their blood glucose responded to the various meals that they ate. The team recorded over 1.5 million glucose readings over the course of the first part of the study.

As they predicted, people had different responses from one another. One food that most of us would associate with a high glycemic response is white bread, and some people did, indeed, have a huge blood glucose spike in response to white bread; however, white bread had almost no effect on the blood glucose response for others.

For every single food tested, they found that some people had a high response to that food, while others had either a medium or low response to that same food. As an example, some people had a high glycemic response to ice cream but a low glycemic response to rice, while others had a high glycemic response to rice and a low glycemic response to ice cream. One big surprise was that ice cream spiked blood glucose in only 35% of participants, while rice spiked blood glucose in 65% of those studied. Yes, much to their surprise, it seems that ice cream wasn't a problem for 65% of those studied!

After these initial tests, they decided to take it one step further and see how they could use this data to give personal dietary recommendations based on specific individual factors. They worked to develop an algorithm that would take these individual differences, including both gut microbiome composition and genetic factors, into account. As an example, they knew that *Actinobacteria* in the gut microbiome is associated with a high glycemic response to both glucose and bread, and both *Proteobacteria* and *Enterobacteriaceae* are associated with overall poor glycemic control and other characteristics of metabolic syndrome, such as obesity and insulin resistance. They used this information plus other data to develop the algorithm.

After developing and then validating the predictive algorithm, it was time for the team to see if their program worked. They created "good" and "bad" diets for 26 new participants, using the predictive algorithm to calculate predicted glucose responses (once again, these predictions were based on personal information from each participant, including the composition of their gut microbiomes and genetic factors).

One example of a "good" diet for a specific participant included: bread and eggs, pita and hummus, edamame, noodles, and ice cream, while the same person's "bad" diet included: muesli (cereal), sushi, marzipan, corn and nuts, and coffee and chocolate. It's interesting to note that some of the items on this participant's "good" list are associated with a higher glycemic index when we look at standardized GI lists. Who would think that bread, pita, noodles, and ice cream would belong on the list of foods that *didn't* cause a big blood glucose response in certain people?

Each of these participants followed their "good" diets for a week and their "bad" diets for a week. The order of the diets was randomized, and participants did not know which diet was the "good" diet and which was the "bad" diet while they were following it.

After analyzing the data, scientists found that just as predicted, the "good" diet resulted in an average lower glucose response when compared to the "bad" diet. In addition, while following the "good" diets, the participants had significantly fewer blood glucose variations. When on the "bad" diets, participants had a typical pre-diabetic blood glucose profile, and while on the "good" diets, they had normal blood glucose control.

One other interesting result was that the participants experienced beneficial changes to their overall gut microbiome composition after following the "good" diets, and they had negative changes following the "bad" diets. This shows that the gut microbiome can change quickly in response to what we are eating.

How can we use this information to help us *Feast Without Fear*? First of all, it validates yet again that we are all different, and so we should be skeptical of any dietary advice that assumes that we all have the same responses to foods.

This information should THRILL you!

To understand that we all respond differently to food is incredibly freeing, because it means that we can forever ignore any one-size-fits-all recommendations and instead focus on how foods make us feel. We also understand that WE didn't fail a particular diet: the diet failed US!

As Dr. Segal mentioned in the video, you can apply this information to measure your own responses to various foods. This would be most beneficial for anyone who suspects that certain foods are a problem for them. After eating any questionable foods, you can test your personal blood glucose response to see if your hunch is correct. This will allow you to identify which foods cause your body to release excess glucose, so that you may avoid them if necessary.

So, you may wonder: am I planning to start testing my blood glucose after every meal? No. I am currently at a normal weight, and I have no risk factors that would indicate that I have issues related to blood glucose control, insulin resistance, or other metabolic issues. However, if you do have these types of health concerns, this may be a valid approach for you. You may be surprised at what you discover about yourself!

Some companies are taking the principles from this research and developing their own predictive algorithms to make personal dietary recommendations to clients. Expect to see this type of service popping up more and more over the coming years. Instead of reading a book that promises to tell you the perfect diet for everyone, you may be equipped, through science, with a personalized nutrition plan tailored just for you: YOUR very own perfect diet. You will simply provide a sample of your DNA and a sample from your gut microbiome, and then receive your own personal dietary recommendations.

Since most of us aren't going to start testing our blood glucose after every meal, and these services are not yet wide spread, is there anything we can do to help us figure out what foods work well for us individually, right now? The answer is yes, and I will talk about that in the next chapter.

Chapter 12

What foods work for you?

While all of my research has pointed me toward an overall template of what may compose an "ideal" diet for most of us, based on traditional foods enjoyed in the Blue Zones, foods that feed our gut microbiomes well, and principles from a Mediterranean-type diet, I have also learned that individual differences are going to play a huge role in how our bodies respond to foods. I shared this with you in previous chapters.

Even though I believe we should not be afraid of any real foods, that does not mean that every person is going to thrive on the same specific foods. We all have unique genetic factors and also different gut microbiomes. Some of us may also have a very unhealthy metabolic profile caused by years of eating the Standard American Diet (also known as "SAD", which I think is accurate.)   The SAD eating pattern isn't good for anyone's gut microbiome or genetic type.

Perhaps if we had never eaten processed and chemically-laden foods, we wouldn't find ourselves in this state. Wouldn't it be nice to travel back in time and tell our 15-year-old selves that we really SHOULD eat more vegetables and avoid junk foods? There are a few other things I would like to tell my 15-year-old self, now that I think about it. I wonder if I would listen to my future self?

Since we can't do that, we each have to start from where we are today, and work with our body's current state, whatever that may be. Someone with Type 2 diabetes is going to have different challenges when compared to someone who is healthy overall, but simply wants to lose a few pounds. Someone who has been overweight for decades is going to face a more difficult struggle than someone who has only recently begun to have a weight problem.

Yes, we have learned that we are all different, and our bodies don't all respond the same way to foods. For that reason, it's important to take all of the food recommendations in this book as a general guide. Someone with a compromised gut microbiome is going to have trouble with foods that others eat freely with no issues.

If you have autoimmune conditions or specific food intolerances, you are going to have to work around any dietary limitations that your body currently faces. That's just a fact. While it may be exciting to think that many people around the world are able to eat all types of foods with no ill effects, some of us are starting from a place of compromised health, and if that is true for you, you are probably going to have to take some basic steps in order to find the type of healing you desire.

The first step is to pay attention to how foods make you feel. I want to tell you a secret about your body: it desperately wants to be healthy. Every choice your body makes behind the scenes (out of your conscious control) is to protect you. The key is to learn how to work *with* your body rather than against it.

One thing about living an intermittent fasting lifestyle is that you may notice right away if a food doesn't work for you. After a period of fasting, you will notice the effects of foods much more dramatically. If any foods you eat make you shaky, give you a stomach ache, or make you want to binge-eat, these are probably not foods that work well for you. As an example, I have learned over time that I personally feel best when I eat a diet that includes lots of carbs and fats from whole foods. I eat plenty of whole grains, potatoes, and vegetables, and fats such as olive oil, butter, and heavy cream. I have learned that I can't open my window with overly refined carbs or anything that is sugary, or I feel shaky. Too much heavy meat makes my stomach hurt, as does a meal heavy in fried foods. I have learned to listen to my body and eat what makes me feel best. Of course, we know that the foods that make me feel best won't necessarily be the ones that make you feel best.

So, the first step is to learn to listen to the way your body feels when you eat. Even though I want you to *Feast Without Fear*, part of that is accepting that you probably won't feast on the same foods that I feast upon, since we are different.

People sometimes misunderstand the advice I give, which is to "eat whatever you want." This doesn't mean that you should eat foods that are problematic for your body. As an example, my son has a shellfish allergy: he can't ever eat shellfish. Instead of literally taking "eat whatever you want" as a command for you to eat all foods, you need to recognize it as permission to eat what you prefer, while still working within your own unique dietary needs.

Going forward, we need to shift our thinking. Rather than classifying foods as "good" or "bad", think about it this way: there are foods that make **you** feel good, and foods that **don't** make you feel good. And, we understand that this will not be the same for each of us.

How do you figure out what foods work best for you? One strategy is to use a food journal to take notes related to what you eat and how you feel. If you are trying to lose weight, see if there are any connections between what you eat and your overall weight loss trends. By doing this, you will most likely be able to figure out what foods work for you over time. Once you do that, you can go on to *Feast Without Fear* forever, making sure to always include foods that feed your gut microbiomes well AND make you feel vibrantly healthy.

However, after paying attention to how foods make you feel, you may suspect that you have specific food intolerances. If so, you may need to take the process one step further. There are many elimination diets out there that you can use to test specific foods and determine how they affect your body. Learning how to use an elimination diet to pinpoint your body's intolerances is beyond the scope of my book, but the good news is that there are already excellent books out there to help you figure it out for yourself. You may have heard of a book called *The Virgin Diet,* or a plan called *Whole 30*. Both of those are elimination diet programs that many people have used successfully to figure out what foods work well for them. I don't endorse either of them specifically, but I have seen people use both of them to identify what dietary changes they need to make.

While I know that it's no fun to think that you may need to eliminate certain foods, it is entirely possible that some foods are not working well in your body at this moment, and we know that this may be related to either your current gut microbiome composition or genetic factors that you aren't aware of. In *The Virgin Diet*, you eliminate 7 common foods that cause problems in many people. Then, you add them back one at a time to see how your body responds. This is a great way to figure out if certain foods cause problems for you. *The Whole 30* plan, which is really popular right now, works in a similar way.

Yes, it is a LOT of work to eliminate foods from your diet temporarily. NO, not one of us wants to imagine that our favorite foods may not work well for us. That being said, figuring out what foods work in your unique body may be the difference between success and failure when it comes to meeting your health and weight loss goals.

If you don't want to rely on a book or a do-it-yourself elimination diet, consider finding a health professional who has experience in this area. Look for a practitioner who practices complementary, alternative, or integrative health to help you work through this process. This webpage from the National Institutes of Health website has information about complementary and integrative health care, and how to find practitioners in your local area:

The bottom line is this: while I don't want anyone to be afraid of any real foods, you may need to face the fact that some foods don't work for you right now, at this point in your life. That doesn't mean that they will never work for you. Through intermittent fasting, we can reverse many of the problems associated with our previous eating habits. By making careful and deliberate food choices, we can slowly rebuild a healthy gut microbiome and begin to heal metabolic issues. At some point, you may be able to reintroduce some or all of the foods that were previously problematic for you.

The best news of all is that we can all make choices today and each and every day that lead us toward a healthier future.

As I said, your plate may not look like mine. The foods that make me feel good may not work at all for you, and vice versa. As you learn to listen to your body, you will see what your body loves, just as I have. Intermittent fasting really teaches us to listen to our bodies, as I already mentioned.

As we work to heal our bodies by eating the foods that make our bodies feel good, it's important for us to understand the difference between "food" and "food-like products." One of these will lead us toward better health over time, and the other will not. I'm sure you know where I am going with this.

Chapter 13

Simple changes that make a big difference

"Food" vs. "Food-like products"

For this chapter, I searched for all research studies that linked highly processed and artificial foods to vibrant health and longevity. Guess what? There are none.

As we learned in the chapter on the gut microbiome, a healthy gut thrives on REAL foods, while growth of an unhealthy gut is encouraged by the intake of overly processed, refined, and artificial foods. So, we now know that eating a diet that contains a lot of highly refined foods, preservatives, and artificial sweeteners creates an unhealthy gut. We also learned that when we have an unhealthy gut microbiome, we are more likely to have unhealthy conditions and illnesses.

As people start to make dietary changes that encourage a healthy gut microbiome, most people find that they actually start to crave healthier foods. As I mentioned in chapter 6, an unhealthy gut sends messages to your brain (thanks to the gut-brain axis) causing you to crave more and more processed and refined foods. As you change your gut, you will probably find that your cravings for these foods diminish.

We also know that intermittent fasting changes your gut microbiome in a positive way. Coupling an intermittent fasting lifestyle with dietary choices that encourage a diverse and healthy gut microbiome is a powerful combination for long-term health.

Change your gut, change your cravings. It's pretty remarkable how that happens over time. As I mentioned in the previous chapter, I have learned that I now feel best on a diet that is high in plant foods. I eat a lot of vegetables, whole grains, starches, and also plenty of fat. It turns out that my body has gravitated naturally to a Mediterranean dietary pattern without me consciously making the decision to do so. I used to eat a lot of fast food, but at some point, my body began to turn away from these types of food-like products. I didn't do this on purpose; it happened naturally. If you had told me three years ago that I would be eating this way, I would not have believed you. I genuinely believe that intermittent fasting has allowed me to get in touch with what foods make me feel best, and as I have made different choices based on that information from my body, I have changed my gut microbiome into one that sends me cravings for zucchini and avocado rather than fast food. I would rather eat beans than filet mignon. I barely recognize myself, frankly.

As we work to cultivate a healthy gut microbiome, we should all have the goal to add more real foods to our plates and replace the food-like products whenever possible. It's actually easier than you might think, and it can be as simple as making a few substitutions at the grocery store.

Recently, I watched a documentary featuring food writer Michael Pollan. The documentary is part of a series called *Cooked,* and it is available on Netflix. The particular episode that caught my attention is called *Air,* and it highlights the importance of bread throughout the world and the traditions surrounding it. I highly recommend this episode, though the others are also interesting. (I would suggest starting with this episode first. *Air* is actually episode 3, but it is my favorite in the series, by far. I also really liked episode 4, which is about fermented foods that are great for our gut microbiomes. Watch episode 3, then episode 4, and if you like them, go back to episodes 1 and 2.)

As I watched that episode with my husband, I thought back to a conversation I had just witnessed in our Facebook intermittent fasting support group. One member was discussing how she had not lost much weight, and was asking for suggestions. In her initial question, she shared that she was a vegetarian who loves bread. Immediately, many group members zeroed in on that statement: "loves bread." The immediate consensus was that she would need to completely give up bread in order to lose any weight. (I did not share in that consensus, by the way.)

As my husband and I watched the episode of *Cooked* together, I mentioned this conversation to him. It's important to note that he has never dieted in his life (though he does now follow an intermittent fasting lifestyle, because he is convinced of the health benefits), so he doesn't have years of dietary dogma to unlearn. He looked at me like I was crazy: people are afraid of bread? Bread is a food that has been instrumental to human survival ever since the first group of people learned how to turn the seed of this grass into a loaf. My husband couldn't even conceive of the notion of being afraid of bread.

As we continued to watch the episode, we saw bread through the eyes of people who depend upon it for their very existence. In one scene, a Moroccan woman mixed flour and water in a big bowl on the floor of her living room while her son watched. She mixed and kneaded, and skillfully assembled the loaf that would become their source of nutrition for the day. As she worked, her words (which were translated from her native language and written as subtitles) resonated with me: "We make bread every morning. Homemade bread is best. It's much better than any bread in the store. You can't live without water, and you can't live without bread. You just can't."

Listen to that again.

"You can't live without water, and you can't live without bread."

Bread is literally the staff of life to her, and to most other cultures all around the world. If there should be a worldwide wheat shortage, people would starve. And yet, here in America and in other countries with a more Western diet, we are so scared of bread that we are cautioning others against eating it. Why is that?

Of course, part of it is because the bread that many of us buy in the stores doesn't resemble the handmade bread carefully crafted there on the living room floor by the woman in Morocco. It's also true that some people do have intolerances related to certain foods, and grains may be one of them. Interestingly, though, many people all over the world eat bread every day with no issues. These people would have no comprehension of what it means to avoid grains or to be "gluten free."

Why do so many people eating a typical Western diet have trouble with bread or other grains? Well, of course, it may be related to the state of our gut microbiomes. If you have a compromised gut, you may find that certain grains are an intolerance for you until you heal your gut. It may also be related to the fact that much of our bread is really a "food-like product" rather than actual "bread."

As I have been researching for and writing this book, I have taken a closer look at many foods in my own kitchen. When I realized the detrimental effect of a diet high in processed foods, chemicals, and preservatives on the overall health of my gut microbiome, I knew I wanted to make a few changes, and one of those changes included the bread that I feed myself and my family. Yes, I eat bread every day of my life, but what bread? While I love to cook, I don't have the time to make my own bread from scratch every day. Is there a way that I could improve the quality of the bread that my family and I eat? The answer, of course, was yes.

I went into my kitchen and read the ingredients on the bread that I served most frequently with dinner. As a habit, I had been purchasing a bag of frozen dinner rolls that only needed about 10 minutes in the oven to be ready for our meal each night. They turned out fluffy and golden, and ready for some butter. Delicious! But, what was in these rolls?

Here's the list of ingredients: *Bleached enriched wheat flour (wheat flour, malted barley flour, niacin, ferrous sulfate, thiamin mononitrate, riboflavin, folic acid), water, sugar, eggs, soybean oil, salt, hydrogenated cottonseed oil, yeast, mono and diglycerides, and whey.*

That isn't too terrible when compared to some other brands of bread available, but if I were planning to mix up some bread dough in my own kitchen, I wouldn't pull out my hydrogenated cottonseed oil and my diclycerides and get busy. That list of ingredients didn't resemble any homemade bread recipe I had ever seen, so I knew I could do better. My gut counted on me.

My next stop was the grocery store. I still wanted to feed bread to my family every night, but I wanted it to be something that more closely resembled actual bread, and not a list of ingredients I wouldn't recognize if they were in front of me. I read the list of ingredients on package after package, and some brands were much worse than the dinner rolls I had in my own freezer. The longer the list, the more "un-foodlike" were the ingredients.

Here's one brand I found, with a list of ingredients that was much worse than the one I had buying: *Enriched flour (wheat flour, malted barley flour, niacin, reduced iron, thiamine mononitrate, riboflavin, folic acid), water, sugar, liquid sugar (sugar, water), butter (pasteurized cream, salt), eggs, contains less than 2 % of each of the following: potato flour, yeast, whey, nonfat milk, soy flour, salt, degerminated yellow corn flour, wheat gluten, sodium stearoyl lactylate, datem, monocalcium phosphate, wheat flour, calcium sulfate, sodium silicoaluminate, ascorbic acid added as a dough conditioner, ammonium sulfate, wheat starch, sorbitan monostearate, enzymes, microcrystalline cellulose, calcium silicate.* That brand definitely didn't make the cut. It sounds more like a chemistry experiment than a loaf of bread.

Finally, I found a brand of frozen bread with these ingredients: *unbleached French wheat flour, water, yeast, salt, ascorbic acid (vitamin C).* Other than the ascorbic acid (vitamin C), every ingredient was something I could envision having at home in my kitchen. I happily purchased that brand of bread, and it has replaced the one with the longer list of ingredients. Guess what? It actually tastes better, too. I toss a couple of these rolls in the oven almost every night to accompany our dinner.

This type of switch is easy to make, and it doesn't require that you give up foods. Instead, you can make a few simple switches that could have a huge impact in the overall quality of what you are consuming.

After all: in today's modern world, it is not practical for most of us to start the day kneading bread dough on our living room floors. We aren't going to be able to prepare every food from scratch using only whole food ingredients. I know this. However, we can become a label reader, and an ingredients snob.

Here is another example of what that looks like in practice. I eat guacamole several times per week. It's one of my favorite foods, in fact. That being said, I don't want to take the time to make it from scratch every time I want to eat it.

One well-known brand of guacamole has this list of ingredients: *Water, Canola Oil, Corn Starch (Modified), Corn Syrup Solids, Crushed Tomatoes (Water, crushed Tomatoes), 2% or less of the following: Whey Protein Concentrate, Salt, Sugar, Dried Onion, Glucono Delta Lactone, Artificial Flavors with Extratives of Paprika (Color), Cultured Cream (Cultured Cream, Skim Milk Powder, Lactic Acid, Xanthan Gum, Potassium Sorbate), Maltodextrin, Garlic Powder, Monosodium Glutamate, Avocado Powder, Dried Red Bell Pepper, Spices, Partially Hydrogenated Soybean Oil, Jalapeno*

*Pepper Powder, Dried Jalapeno Pepper, Citric Acid, Lemon Juice
Solids, Caramel Color, Soy Sauce (Fermented Wheat, Soybeans,
Salt, Maltodextrin, Caramel Color), Yellow 5 (Water, FD&C
Yellow 5, Sodium Benzoate, Phosphoric Acid), Sodium Acid
Pyrophosphate, DATEM, Lactic Acid, Xanthan Gum, Locust Bean
Gum, FD&C Blue.*

Does that look like guacamole you would make in
your kitchen? No, it doesn't resemble any guacamole recipe I
have ever seen. Can you imagine yourself preparing it?
Hmmm, I think it needs just one more dash of locust bean
gum and another pinch of maltrodextin. I believe I'll add a
little more monosodium glutamate. Pass the glucano delta
lactone, please. Uh, no thank you.

Instead, I buy the brand that lists these ingredients:
*Haas avocados, tomatoes, red onions, onions, jalapeno peppers,
cilantro, lime juice, sea salt, garlic.* If I were going to make
homemade guacamole, those are exactly the ingredients I
would assemble.

The best news of all is that the brands with the fewer
ingredients actually taste better. Of course, the bad news is
that they are usually more expensive. Since I live an
intermittent fasting lifestyle, I am now completely willing to
pay more for foods of higher quality. If I am only eating one
main meal per day, it is going to be the best quality food that
I can find. My body deserves it, and so does yours. I also
think of the money I save by not driving through a fast food
restaurant to pick up breakfast every morning like I used to
do. Yes, I can pay a little more for high quality bread and
the better tasting guacamole made from real ingredients
rather than the one that resembles a chemistry experiment.

Take a tour of the grocery store for yourself. For any
item you want to purchase, don't just grab the brand you
usually buy and throw it into your cart. Instead, take a look
at all of the brands surrounding it. Read the lists of
ingredients. How does your normal brand compare? It's
easy to go for the option with the shortest list of ingredients,
and the ones that most resemble "food" rather than "food-

like chemicals." You'll be surprised at how easy it is to make this simple switch. The closer your food is to "food" rather than "food-like products", the easier it is to *Feast Without Fear*.

Before I go on, I need to take a moment to caution you about taking this practice too far. We can get so caught up in "food perfection" that we are afraid to eat foods that don't meet our new rigorous standards of quality. That is not my goal with this chapter. I want you to *Feast Without Fear*, and not live your life paralyzed with anxiety about every bite you eat.

Somewhere between "total crap junk food of whatever you can find" and "all natural organic unprocessed food perfection" is your unique sweet spot. You have to experiment to find what works best for you and makes you feel good. If you are having trouble meeting your health and weight loss goals, move closer to the all-natural, organic, and unprocessed side of the spectrum. In the real world, though, who wants to give up everything? Not me. I don't fill the majority of my diet with processed junk foods, but I can eat some of these foods alongside higher quality choices and still feel healthy. I have found a balance that works well for me.

So, instead of feeling like you need to be absolutely flawless when it comes to your food, make small changes that support your health goals. It may help if I share some good news about how small changes add up in a big way. In July of 2017, a study called *Association of Changes in Diet Quality with Total and Cause-Specific Mortality* was published. I am giving you a link to the abstract only, because that is all that is available without a subscription:

http://www.nejm.org/doi/full/10.1056/NEJMoa161 3502

In this study, researchers analyzed results from over 73,000 participants, whose dietary quality was reported over a 12-year period. This included 47,994 women from the

Nurses' Health Study and 25,745 men from the Health Professionals Follow-Up Study.

Scientists tracked overall changes in each participant's "diet quality" by using several eating rating scales. They found that for every 20-percentile increase in a participant's diet score, which indicated that the participant was making positive dietary changes, there were significant reductions in overall mortality. This illustrates that every positive change we make can have an impact. Here, even small dietary changes were linked to a reduced risk of death.

Based on this information, we can feel good about every small change we ourselves make, while releasing the burden we might otherwise place on our shoulders to meet some sort of unrealistic dietary perfection. Here's how I make this work for my lifestyle. When I have a choice, I always choose the highest quality option available to me at the time. That's it—it really is that simple. Many of the foods I eat do have processed ingredients, and it's okay.

If we are choosing a good number of high-quality foods every day, and we are feeding our gut microbiomes well over time, we can still enjoy other foods from time to time, or even every day. If most of your plate contains real and high-quality foods, don't panic over the few suspect ingredients in your bottle of salad dressing, or worry about the ice cream treat you go get with your kids. Perfection is not possible or even desired. We are looking for a healthy lifestyle, and worrying obsessively about every food you eat is also not going to be healthy.

Make it a goal to include as many healthy foods as you can, switch to brands with fewer ingredients when possible, and don't worry about the few less-than-perfect ingredients or foods that you want to enjoy. Sometimes I'm going to eat a hot dog from Costco, and it's not going to destroy my health in one meal. The overall pattern of what you eat is much more important than any one ingredient, meal, or indulgence. Find a balance.

So: what foods do we want to make sure to include more of in our diets? In the next chapter, I am going to pull all of the recommendations into one place.

Chapter 14

Foods to feast upon without fear

Are you ready for some good news/bad news? Here it is: I am not going to give you a meal plan to follow. YOU are going to have to figure out what foods work best for your unique body, and I can't tell you exactly what that will look like for you.

This is the moment where some people may start to get nervous. I can hear it now:

Wait, Gin. Are you telling me that you are NOT going to give me a 21-day meal plan? Where are the lists of foods that are "allowed" and foods that are "forbidden"? Can I eat dessert / potatoes / carbs / bacon / bread / pizza / _____ (fill in the blank)??? HELP!!!!! WHAT EXACTLY AM I SUPPOSED TO EAT?!?!?!?!?

Isn't that how diet books work? The author gives you the background information, and then tells you exactly what diet you are now expected to follow. Everything is spelled out for you, easy-peasy. Armed with a grocery list of "approved" foods, you head out to begin your new life, on this new diet.

Well, the body isn't easy-peasy. As I have reiterated throughout the book, everyone's body is different.

Also, this isn't a diet book. Consider this an ANTI-diet book, in fact.

As we discussed in the last chapter, we want to make sure that we are eating a higher proportion of actual "foods" instead of "food-like products." When in doubt, err on the side of real foods. On the other hand, eat cake if you are celebrating. You have to figure out the balance that works for you.

Your overall goal is to create an enjoyable lifestyle that includes all of the foods that you love and that make you feel vibrantly healthy. While it is important to exclude any foods that don't work well for you, it's easy to select delicious foods that make you feel great, all without worrying about the calorie count or the specific macronutrient ratios.

Even though we understand that all of us are unique, and therefore foods will work differently in our bodies, we can still consider an overall template of healthy choices that will work for most of us. As we learn to *Feast Without Fear*, we can take lessons from the three sources that I mentioned in chapters 5-8: the Blue Zones, our gut microbiomes, and the well-researched Mediterranean-type dietary pattern. I am putting all of these recommendations here, in three lists. Take the suggestions from these lists as an overall template of what promotes longevity and health, including a diverse and robust gut microbiome.

Of course, take your own individual responses to foods into account. If you know you are lactose intolerant, don't pick dairy foods. If you have Celiac disease, you aren't going to be able to eat foods with gluten. Remember: there are NO one-size-fits-all dietary recommendations. Go back to chapter 12 if you need help figuring out what foods from these lists work best for you and your unique body.

Now, let's look at the lists that will make up our overall healthy eating template. Notice the similarities between the lists, and think about which foods sound delicious to you. Start with those. Make your own grocery lists and food plan crafted around what you **want** to eat.

What do people eat in the Blue Zones?

As we read in chapter 5, some of the longest living people in the world live in what Dan Buettner and his team of scientists have named the Blue Zones. Because these people live in different countries—Greece, Italy, Japan, Costa Rica, and the United States—they all have different local foods available to them. Even so, they all have certain things in common. Their diets all follow basic guidelines, which we can incorporate. To eat like residents of the Blue Zones:

- Don't count calories or restrict entire groups of macronutrients.

- Enjoy the foods that you eat, and stop when you have had enough.

- Include a wide variety of carbohydrates, proteins, and fats, with no conscious restrictions in any category.

- Focus a large proportion of your daily intake on foods from plant sources, including: beans, leafy greens, vegetables, fruits, nuts, and whole grains.

- Enjoy meat and use dairy products, based on your preferences, but not necessarily with every meal or even every day.

- Limit overly processed/refined foods and sugary foods.

- Drink coffee, tea, water, and a moderate amount of alcohol, according to your lifestyle preferences. (Of course, all of these beverage choices are optional. Don't select beverages that don't work for you, just as you shouldn't select foods that don't work for you.)

Which foods feed our gut microbiomes well?

In chapter 6, we learned how important it is to feed our gut microbiomes well. So much of our own personal health relies on keeping this community of bacteria happy and diverse. Fortunately, we have learned that we can structure our diets to ensure that we are feeding our guests well:

- Eat foods that are high in MACs, or Microbiota Accessible Carbohydrates. These include: unrefined whole grains, vegetables, legumes (beans), and fruits.

- Choose foods that are high in inulin, which are prebiotic foods. Some of these include: garlic, leeks, onion, bananas, wheat bran, wheat flour, nuts, and asparagus.

- Select resistant starches. Note that one of the best ways to make your starches "more resistant" is to cook and then cool them. Green bananas are also a good source of resistant starch.

- Eat foods high in phytonutrients (natural plant chemicals). These are found in various colored vegetables and fruits ("eat the rainbow": red, orange, yellow, green, blue, and purple). Phytonutrients are also found in some of our favorites: cocoa, wine, tea, and coffee.

- Include probiotic foods. These include: yogurt, kefir, kimchi, sauerkraut, apple cider vinegar, and certain cheeses (not the overly processed "cheese food" versions).

- Avoid overly processed or refined foods, since they feed the "bad guys" in our gut, which then crowd out the "good guys".

What is a typical "Mediterranean Dietary Pattern"?

In chapter 8, we learned that the Mediterranean dietary pattern is associated with many positive health outcomes, based on much of the evidence from various scientific studies. While you may not live in a Mediterranean climate, there are certain characteristics that make up this Mediterranean dietary pattern:

- Eat a wide variety of fruits and vegetables.

- Use olive oil as a main source of dietary fat, but include other sources of real-food fats, such as those from dairy products.

- Choose whole grain products, including bread, pasta, rice, and other cereal foods.

- Enjoy beans and nuts.

- Select dairy products, including natural cheeses.

- Enjoy fish, and also meat (in moderation).

- Beverages may include water, tea, coffee, and moderate alcohol (specifically red wine). (As I already mentioned, select beverages that fit into your specific lifestyle preferences.)

- Avoid overly refined or processed foods.

As you look over these three lists, you should notice that they are very similar. In fact, I have already mentioned these similarities several times throughout the chapters of this book. When we notice that people in the Blue Zones are eating foods that are great for promoting diversity and health in our gut microbiomes, and that the Mediterranean diet, one of the most well-researched and recommended dietary patterns, also includes these very same foods, it paints a compelling picture of an overall dietary template that we can use to craft our own individual dietary plans.

Our goal should be to select liberally from these lists, while paying attention to how foods make us feel. Make choices based on the foods you enjoy and how you want to live your life.

Besides foods, are there any other factors that help us live a longer and healthier life? The answer is, of course, yes.

Chapter 15

Vibrant health: More than just *what* you eat

We know that it's important to make dietary choices that support healthy outcomes. From intermittent fasting to feeding our gut microbiomes, when and what we eat both make a big difference in our overall health.

We are more than just food-digesters, however. As humans, we are emotional creatures, and it's important to take care of both our bodies and our minds.

When we look at the Blue Zones, we can make a list of what they are eating; but we can't completely separate the effects of foods from overall lifestyle choices. The same can be said for the Mediterranean dietary recommendations. It's not just "food"; it's also the lifestyle.

One of the papers I linked in chapter 8 had a "Mediterranean Diet Pyramid" in Figure 5. That pyramid can be found at this link:

https://www.ncbi.nlm.nih.gov/pmc/articles/PMC4222885/pdf/12916_2014_Article_994.pdf .

When you look at the base of the pyramid, they list several lifestyle factors that have nothing to do with what we eat. These include: regular physical activity, sufficient rest, and something they call "conviviality." What is conviviality? It's defined by Miriam-Webster (online) as *"relating to, occupied with, or fond of feasting, drinking, and good company."*

That actually sounds like they are telling us to *Feast Without Fear*; am I right? Bring on the conviviality!

Besides just eating foods that support health, we must make sure to take care of our other physical and emotional needs. Surround ourselves with a community made up of friends and family. Get plenty of sleep. Play hard. Love your life, in every way you can.

Easier said than done, perhaps? Maybe. But just as in making food choices that support vibrant health, we can also make lifestyle choices that allow us to de-stress.

I mentioned a couple of books in previous chapters that I highly recommend, and I want to mention them again: *Super Genes: Unlock the Astonishing Power of your DNA for Optimum Health and Well* Being, by Rudolph Tanzi and Deepak Chopra, and *Thrive: Finding Happiness the Blue Zones Way*, by Dan Buettner. Both of these books give you practical suggestions for improving your life in meaningful ways, beyond just dietary choices.

As you work on enhancing your lifestyle in non-food related ways, you still may be tempted from time to time to fall into the old patterns of "diet thinking" from years past. Can we figure out a way to eliminate this particular stress from our lives, forever? The answer is a resounding YES!

Chapter 16

Ignoring dietary noise

I've been a part of the world of competing dietary dogma for a long time. First, as a serial dieter in search of the "perfect" plan that would tell me exactly what foods to eat and what foods to avoid. None of those plans ever worked for me, because I was relying on someone else to tell me exactly what to eat.

Now, I see this world of dietary dogma in my role as an administrator of two intermittent fasting support groups on Facebook. As of the fall of 2017, we have over 37,000 members combined in the groups I moderate, and we continue to grow quickly as IF spreads and becomes mainstream. Because we don't promote any one style of eating, group members are both free and encouraged to find their own best plans.

New members (and even long-term members) frequently have very specific views on how they (and everyone else) should eat in order to have best results. I have noticed one thing that is almost universal. When you find someone who does well on a particular eating regimen, they are often very earnest that their plan is the best plan for everyone. They can point you to doctors who support it. They are armed with documentaries, YouTube links, and TedTalks about their eating plan, and they also love to post links to scientific studies that support their preferred approach.

Here's something else about followers of this type of dietary dogma: they believe that because they feel so much better on their plan, that you would too. If you tell them that you tried it and you didn't feel well eating that way, they will reply that you must have done it wrong. You must not have eaten the right combination of foods; otherwise you would have loved it, just as they do. If you had only done it correctly, you would feel better, just like them.

After reading this book, I want one thing for you: I want you to be able to ignore all of this dietary noise. I want you to ignore any documentary that says there is "one true way." Ignore people who say that their diet is "better." They don't live in your body.

It's also best to avoid arguments with others about what you should be eating. Don't be tempted to get into a "my study is better than your study" duel. If you want to find studies and diet books that show one way of eating is the best, you can do it. If you want to find studies and diet books that show the complete opposite way of eating is the best, you can do that, too.

What's interesting is that we have members who are finding success using every possible approach to eating that exists. People are thriving on a low-fat plant-based approach. Others are thriving on a high-fat no-grain approach. Insert literally any dietary approach here, and I can find someone who is finding success with it.

Now that we have learned that our bodies really are all unique, thanks to the genetic factors that shape us upon birth and the individual gut microbiomes that reside within us, we know that there really is no such thing as a one-size-fits-all plan.

Because we understand this, we must stop going to others for recommendations about what we ourselves should eat. Overall, we should stop putting the blame on single macronutrients like carbs, protein, or fat, and look at food holistically. Within our bodies, foods work synergistically, rather than in isolation.

We are finally free to ignore what other people say about how foods make *them* feel. Understand that every expert who writes a diet book legitimately feels better eating that way, but that doesn't mean YOU will. Your gut is different. Your genes are different.

We are finally free to ignore any overly simplistic set of dietary guidelines based on a single factor, such as "carbs: bad." Be cautious when you hear all-or-nothing statements, such as these:

- No one should eat grains.
- Everyone should eat grains.

Both of those statements are too broad to be true. There are many people around the world who thrive while eating grains, and there are also people who have problems related to grain consumption.

After all of my research and studying over the past years, particularly the targeted studying I have done over the past few months, I've come to a conclusion about all of the diet war food-noise.

I'm done. And it is absolutely breathtakingly freeing.

All of my research on genetic differences, the gut microbiome, and the Blue Zones has convinced me that we can make ourselves insane by combing PubMed for studies about perfect diets. We can watch documentary after documentary, and YouTube video after YouTube video, becoming more and more confused about what to eat. We can follow expert after expert, who all have science-y claims that back up what they are saying.

Or, we can take a lesson from the longest living people in the world. We can eat foods that taste good. We can learn to listen to our bodies and feed ourselves a wide variety of nutritious foods. We can stop eating foods that we don't feel well eating, and select foods that make us feel vibrant and healthy. Instead of looking for food groups to eliminate based on the dietary trend-du-jour, we can feed our bodies (and our gut microbiomes) a wide variety of delicious foods, full of the nutrients our bodies need.

It's going to be tough, because every day, the dietary noise is going to try to sneak back in.

Learn how to turn off the outside noise and go within. Eat real food that makes you feel good. Avoid foods that make you feel bad. Listen to your body and enjoy your life.

Feast Without Fear.

Appendix A: Recommended reading

I hope that this book has made you "hungry" for more! (See what I did there?) If any of the topics in this book piqued your interest, you'll want to continue your reading by picking up some of these recommended books. All of them should be available through your favorite online or local booksellers.

I have organized this list by topic. Within each topic, books are ranked in order of my "most recommended" to "also recommended."

Food:

As you know, I believe in the power of real food, as opposed to food-like products. While I do still include food-like products in my day-to-day diet, most of the foods that I choose are high quality foods. These books explain how real foods are superior to food-like products, and why it is important to include real foods in our diets.

In Defense of Food: An Eater's Manifesto, **by Michael Pollan** I love this book, and I absolutely love Michael Pollan, too. Perhaps one reason I love it so much is the fact that it's written by a journalist, and not a doctor or nutritionist. Like me, he set out to figure out what we all "should" be eating. Perhaps "normal" non-medical people (like Michael Pollan and me) have an advantage, because we don't have deeply ingrained medical dogma to unlearn. His famous manifesto is simple: *"Eat food. Not too much. Mostly plants."* Based on everything I have learned about the Blue Zones, our gut microbiome, and the research on the benefits of a Mediterranean eating

ern, I believe he is right. Also, you can see that
rmittent fasting fits well within that manifesto,
in the "not too much" guideline.

The Obesity Code, by Jason Fung This is the only book that
is special enough to be recommended in both this
book and my first one, *Delay, Don't Deny*. Even
though I was already at my goal weight when I first
read it, I learned so much about how the body works
within its pages. In this book, Dr. Fung explains the
hormonal imbalances at the root of the modern-day
obesity epidemic, and tells us what we can do about
it. He even convinced me of the importance of
keeping insulin low during the fast, which compelled
me to give up my beloved stevia, and begin fasting
clean. What a difference that makes! As for the most
important takeaway when it comes to what to eat:
choose "real" foods over processed foods for better
health outcomes. Even though Dr. Fung is well-
known for being a low-carb/high-fat (LCHF)
advocate, and he promotes a LCHF way of eating
with many of his patients (particularly those with
Type 2 diabetes), you don't finish *The Obesity Code*
with the thought that carbohydrates are "bad." In
fact, he has a whole chapter of the book devoted to
carbohydrates, and in it, he outlines the protective
properties of the fiber within these foods. He says (on
page 179) that "observational studies consistently
demonstrate that whole grains are protective against
obesity and diabetes." Even with a sentence like that,
some people believe Dr. Fung is completely anti-carb,
which always makes me wonder if they actually read
the same *Obesity Code* that I read.

The Science of Skinny Cookbook, by Dee McCaffrey I
recommended Dee McCaffrey's first book (*The Science
of Skinny*) in *Delay Don't Deny*, and I am
recommending her follow-up cookbook in this one.
As I said in my comments about her first book in
Delay, Don't Deny: I don't agree with her advice to eat
frequent meals throughout the day…obviously.

#IntermittentFastingForTheWin. However, I do agree that she is onto something with her food recommendations. Everything you need to know about choosing real foods is summarized in the first chapter of her cookbook. She explains some of the problems with eating a diet high in refined foods and artificial ingredients. In the second chapter, she outlines the benefits to be found with real and unprocessed foods. The rest of the book is a collection of recipes highlighting the types of foods she recommends. Now that I am an intermittent faster, I enjoy cooking delicious meals made with REAL foods, like the ones found in this cookbook. I can *Feast Without Fear* every single night, selecting delicious foods that are both satisfying and healthy.

The Gut Microbiome:

The books on this list were written by doctors and researchers who are experts on an ideal gut microbiome. In each one, the authors share how they themselves eat. Who better to emulate than someone who understands the gut, literally inside and out?

The Diet Myth: The Real Science Behind What We Eat, **by Tim Spector** This is such a fascinating book, and I have highlighted and tabbed many sections within it. This is the kind of book I plan to read and reread over the years, and each time I do, I get something else out of it. Tim Spector is a professor and researcher, and his main areas of interest are genetics and the gut microbiome. Currently, he is the lead investigator of the British Gut Project. The book is written in the first person, so it isn't a dry and overly scientific book; and even though it is heavy on the science, it's as if he is telling you a very interesting story. I'm pretty sure that I learned something new on every page. Throughout the book, he teaches us about how various foods affect our bodies, with an emphasis on how they affect our gut microbiomes. After reading his book, you will understand, as I do, that we really can *Feast Without Fear*, as long as we feed our

131

microbiomes well! There are times when the book seems to jump from topic to topic almost at random, but because it is just so interesting, I didn't mind.

***The Clever Guts Diet: How to Revolutionise Your Body from the Inside Out*, by Michael Mosley** This book was released in the summer of 2017, and I got my hands on the British version, which is the title I am sharing here. The American version is actually called *The Clever Gut Diet*, but I find the British title to be more charming, so that is the one I went with. (Plus, I haven't read the American version.) This is a very simple book, and isn't nearly as science-y as *The Diet Myth*. The book is divided into two parts. The first part is an introduction to the gut microbiome, and why we care so much about it (which you should already understand, after reading my book.) The second part is called "How to Reboot your Biome—a 2-stage Healing Programme," and I mainly shared that because I just wanted to type "programme" (why is the British spelling always more fun?) All kidding aside, this book gives practical suggestions for what you can do to heal your gut microbiome. Since Michael Mosely is a doctor, you can feel good about taking medical advice from him (rather than me).

***PREbiotics, Not Probiotics*, by Frank Jackson** This book was written by a gastroenterologist, and it's the first book I read that explained the importance of the microbiome. I want to warn you: Dr. Jackson wants to sell you his own line of prebiotic supplement, so he talks about it throughout the book. Even if you aren't interested in his product line, this book gives you the basics about why prebiotics (specifically prebiotic foods) are key when we want to enhance out gut health. He also explains the best way to include these foods in your diet.

The Good Gut: Taking Control of Your Weight, Your Mood, and Your Long-term Health, **by Justin Sonnenburg and Erica Sonnenburg** The Sonnenburgs are a husband and wife duo from Stanford University. This book is not as engaging as some of the other books I have listed, but it is packed with science about our gut microbiomes. I almost didn't include it, but if you are fascinated by the gut microbiome and can't get enough, then add this one to your list.

Blue Zones:

These books are all by the same author, but they each have a different focus. Choose the one that most matches your specific interests—or, read them all! Like Michael Pollan, Dan Buettner is a journalist who wanted to discover the secrets of health and longevity. What he (along with a team of researchers) found is outlined in these books.

The Blue Zones Solution, **by Dan Buettner** If you only want to read one book about the Blue Zones, this is a good one. In part one, Dan introduces you to the five Blue Zones, and explains how the people within these areas live, and even more importantly, how they eat. In part two, he shares how they are taking the lessons from the Blue Zones into other communities to see if they can affect health outcomes within these communities. In part three, he explains how to apply the lessons from the Blue Zones to your own life: both in regard to foods you choose and other lifestyle habits.

The Blue Zones: 9 Lessons for Living Longer from the People Who've Lived the Longest, **by Dan Buettner** This is the original, and gives you an in-depth background of each of the Blue Zones, plus the lessons you can learn from each of them.

Thrive: Finding Happiness the Blue Zones Way, **by Dan Buettner** Yet another book in the Blue Zones series. This book focuses on 4 different communities from around the world: not the longevity Blue Zones, but instead profiles the four "happiest" places on earth, and what we can learn from each of them.

Genes/Epigenetics:

I only have one book listed in this section, but it's a great one.

Super Genes: Unlock the Astonishing Power of your DNA for Optimum Health and Well Being, **by Rudolph Tanzi and Deepak Chopra** This is an eye-opening book, and well worth your time…if you are ready to open your mind to the latest research on genes and epigenetics. Written collaboratively by a physician and a professor of neurology, this book explains how genes are not our fixed destiny, as we have mistakenly believed for so long. We can make choices that affect our gene activity, and through these choices, we can steer this activity in a positive direction. Our genes actually react to our experiences. Some of the practices in the book, such as incorporating medication, may seem to venture away from mainstream medical advice and into the new-age arena; however, the more I read about how the body works, the more I understand that we are a lot more than just a big skin-sack filled with body parts. If you are ready to think about your body-mind connection in a new way, this is a great place to start.

Appendix B: Personal stories

Intermittent fasting continues to change lives, and all over the world, people are learning to *Feast Without Fear* as they successfully implement an intermittent fasting lifestyle. In this section, some of the members of my intermittent fasting support groups have shared how intermittent fasting has affected them, and also how they choose to eat.

I'll be honest: this is my favorite part of the book. As you read these stories, notice how every person has modified and adjusted their IF regimens and food intake to match what makes them feel best. These stories illustrate the message of this book: there truly is NO one-size-fits-all way to eat.

Jessica:

> My life has drastically changed since I began IF. Aside from losing 40 lbs. in 3.5 months, I have more energy for my children, I sleep better, and I feel more confident with my (shrinking) body. I do not eat fast food any longer as I do not have any interest in processed junk, and my mental clarity had improved beyond what I ever could have imagined!

> Before IF I did not eat well. I rarely craved healthy foods. I ate out most days at fast food places and never really enjoyed food. Now my diet consists of really whatever I am in the mood for, between chicken, beef, fish, healthy carb options, and lots of vegetables that I truly enjoy, as well as bread and pasta--without the guilt! I do eat my occasional sweets, but I rarely crave them. Before I found this lifestyle, I would eat cakes and sweets most nights! I

do eat a good amount of butter which is great, because who doesn't love butter!

Tammie, from Ferris, TX:

So far, my journey with intermittent fasting is healing my gut and also healing my unhealthy relationship with food. It has given me so much freedom with food. I no longer feel like a slave, constantly thinking about or daydreaming about my next "date" with food. When I ate, it was never as wonderful as my daydreams were. Now I don't even think about what I'm going to eat! When I'm hungry and my window is open, I listen to my body and eat what I want to eat. The weight loss I have had is slower than most but I know my body is healing from the inside out. The weight loss is a wonderful side effect and I'm looking forward to the rest of my journey!

When I first started intermittent fasting, I went crazy with all the "bad" food I could shove into my mouth in my 4-hour window. Now I'm quite a bit more picky about what I eat. I tend to lean toward eating whole foods and make everything from scratch. I use natural sweeteners when I bake and wholesome ingredients! Due to my husband's medical background and the amount of medication he takes, he is not fasting with me, but he completely supports me and absolutely loves the home cooking! We have some good southern meals like breaded pork chops, mashed potatoes, gravy, and green beans. We love meatloaf and we love our Taco Tuesdays. We also love homemade chili and cornbread with lots of butter. We eat big salads with tons of veggies, fruit, nuts, seeds and dressing. I love the freedom to eat what my body is craving and feel no guilt about blissful indulgences, whether it is simply chocolate or a wonderfully complicated dessert. This way of eating is what I have been looking for my whole adult life!

I am just so thankful that this is not a diet and that I am finally shedding the diet mentality that has consumed me for the last 40 years.

Lisa Simpson:

I began One Meal a Day (OMAD) in January of 2017, at a weight of 172 (180 was my highest weight ever). As of July 2017, my lowest has been 146. I've gone down 3 or 4 sizes depending on the clothes. I'm sleeping better, I have more energy and a LOT more confidence. I think in some ways, I used my weight to keep people away. I'd tell myself, only when I'm thin, then I can....and basically put my life on hold, blaming my unhappiness on my weight. I've struggled with bulimia almost my whole adult life. I felt there were "good" and "bad" food. When I ate the good, I was ok. If I ate the bad, I would get an overwhelming urge to purge it. If I tried to restrict what I ate, I'd obsess over the forbidden foods and quickly fall off whatever diet I was attempting. With IF, nothing is restricted, I'm just delaying when I eat. I can honestly say I feel free of this eating disorder now - for 6 months - and THAT is reason enough to keep with OMAD for life. Food Freedom!

I have NO food restrictions, just delayed gratification. I had already made a lot of dietary changes prior to IF to eat more whole foods, less sugar, less bread and pasta. I love vegetables - I roast them a lot with spices and nutritional yeast. A big salad with lots of different things on it (vegetables, beans, seeds, fruit) makes me happy. I read labels and stay away from anything with added sugar (so unnecessary - why add sugar to tomato sauce?) My meal is usually lots of vegetables, some lean protein (shrimp, fish, chicken) and good fats (avocados, olives, cheese, butter!) In staying away from processed food, I'm cooking a lot more and experimenting with foods and recipes I may not have tried in the past. And then, every once in a while, I'll have a good burger and fries or Chicago deep-dish pizza! The amazing part is there's no more guilt over that!

My advice is to trust the process of IF/OMAD. I didn't lose anything per the scale for the first three weeks but I could see my belly shrinking and clothes fit better. Take measurements to help you keep motivated. Put the scale away. If I compare my "measly" 26 pounds lost to some of the other quick success stories, I'd be discouraged, but seeing the changes in how clothes fit is everything I need!

CJ:

I have lost 5 pounds and I no longer obsess over food. I had gained 15 pounds in the last 3 years, and realized that if I didn't get a grip on my eating food for comfort I was going to be very unhealthy. I also have a circulation disorder in my legs and was experiencing a lot of leg pain. I had tried everything: counting calories, Whole 30, and even an appetite suppressant drink. I could not get a grip! I'm also in my mid-fifties and am going through menopause. One Meal a Day (OMAD) helped me to completely forget about food except for when I have my eating window. This way of eating has taken away my leg pains (because I think my body can now focus on healing), has lessened my hot flashes tremendously, and I can now get a good night's sleep. I'm hooked for life!

I mostly eat a vegetarian diet. I do eat fish and I try to enjoy something sweet every day. I don't want to feel deprived in any way. I like a soda occasionally and always try to open my window with a green smoothie so that I can get plenty of greens. I love to cook but try to make good choices when I do. I eat lots of beans and potatoes.

I love the book (*Delay, Don't Deny*) and appreciate so much this lifestyle, and I'm hoping and praying that my example will rub off on my family members and my friends.

Nick Townsend:

I have lost 25 lbs. and have kept it off. I have also reversed a diagnoses of severe sleep apnea. I have hypothyroidism and my thyroid is working better, requiring a lower dose of medication. My asthma has all but been eliminated; I have come off my steroid inhaler and haven't needed my rescue inhaler in nearly five months.

I have been vegetarian since 2008 and most meals I prepare are actually vegan; this is an extremely personal choice and I would never wish to impose my choice on anyone else. Recently I discovered I had a gut microbiome imbalance and have diligently been using prebiotics and probiotics to repair the damage. In the process, I have discovered that I am no longer craving a lot of sugar and processed carbs but choosing fresh, whole foods. Zucchini noodles with mushrooms, veggie stir fry, sweet potatoes and banana smoothies all are items I consume with delight. PB&J's are also a favorite along with pizza and gelato. I try to keep my unhealthier choices to once a week as I have learned that too much sugar and processed carbs can cause fatigue, brain fog and malaise.

Karin from St. Louis:

I am 43 years old and I have been practicing IF since February 27th of 2017. I will do this for the rest of my life, and I write these words with joy, not resignation. Although I have been losing weight very slowly since I began IF, averaging about 3 lbs. per month, it has been truly life-changing. I have lost weight multiple times in my life via calorie restriction and exercise, but as soon as I stopped counting every calorie that passed my lips, I would inevitably regain. I could never eat like a "normal person." It was so frustrating to watch skinny people eat large amounts of whatever foods they wanted, while I gained 5 pounds just thinking about eating something rich and delicious. I'm a foodie. I really love cooking, baking, coming up with my own recipes, as well as visiting all different kinds of restaurants with dishes from countries around the world. In short: I love food. So, when I realized that, after age 40, I could either be thin and fit OR enjoy food, I was devastated. Then, I read Gin's book *Delay Don't Deny*. Honestly, I didn't fully believe it would work for me, but, the science was there, the testimonials were there, and I was so filled with hope that I tried it. And it worked! I ate literally whatever I wanted, but within a window, and I lost weight instead of gaining.

In the beginning, I ate pizza, cookies, cakes, chips, dips, fast food, etc. Everything I had been depriving myself of, I ate in abundance, and I continued to lose weight without counting calories or doing any sort of exercise at all. Amazing! If we had a social event, I kept my window open longer and I even had a few days here and there where I didn't even fast but ate "normally" all day long. (I felt like garbage the next day of course.)

Then after the first few weeks, I still ate whatever I wanted, but I was no longer craving all the junk food. I still wanted rich, fatty foods and desserts, but I noticed that heavily processed, packaged foods became completely unsatisfying. I ordered some Girl Scout cookies from a friend's child and didn't even eat them. I tried one and threw it away after just one bite. All I could taste were chemicals and fake flavorings; yuck!

One day, I realized that the edema in my legs was gone. I had been experiencing pitted edema in my legs for the past 3 years, and it had completely cleared up. I don't remember exactly when it cleared up, but I believe it was 2 or 3 weeks into fasting. It has never returned. My heartburn is also gone. I was experiencing heartburn on a daily basis, every time I ate, even if I ate healthy foods and small amounts. Now, I never get heartburn. The pain in the arches of my feet has also gone away. The pain in my back has lessened, but it's still there. I still have around 60 lbs. more to lose, so I believe that will get better once I get closer to my goal weight. I have so much more energy throughout the day, even if I haven't gotten a good night's sleep. Add to that another bonus benefit: I don't have to worry about buying and preparing any food to bring with me to work, so I save time and money too! This has been a real game-changer for me.

I still crave pizza, sweets and junk food sometimes, but it has to be truly wonderful pizza, cake, etc. I also find myself craving fruits, veggies and whole foods and rejecting anything that is from a box or package. I have been a vegetarian since I was 8 years old, vegan on and off again for the last 5 years (for the animals, not for health or weight loss), and I am currently eating a pretty high fat, high carb diet. I eat whole foods MOST of the time, but if I want bread and butter, cake, cookies, pizza, chips, dips, etc., I eat them. I don't deny myself anything or feel guilty about eating any more. I eat until I feel full and satisfied.

I finally enjoy eating again and I feel peaceful about food. I eat usually between 3 pm and 8 pm during the work week. Sometimes a snack and dinner, and sometimes my window is only open for an hour or less and I eat only dinner. Snacks are usually pistachios, string cheese and a kombucha. Dinners are always different and either vegan or vegetarian: curried red lentils, carrots and greens in coconut milk served over rice, Frito Pie (vegetarian chili topped with sour cream, cheese, avocado, salsa and corn chips), General Tso's Tofu and veggies with rice noodles, roasted asparagus, garlic rosemary smashed potatoes, dark green salads with sunflower seeds, feta, dried cranberries and either homemade dressing or my favorite store bought one (Pasta House). Desserts are usually homemade cookies, cakes and pies or fresh berries. I often have a glass of red wine or two in my window. If there's a party or any kind of special occasion, I eat and drink as I please that day or have a longer window. (Read: 2 bottles of wine, chips, dips, grazing the whole day.) Basically, I eat my favorite foods every day!

Do I have anything else to add? Yes! An emphatic THANK-YOU to Gin! I have read so many other books about diet, nutrition, fasting, etc.; many of which she recommended, some that she didn't, some I read before, but it was her words that made everything click for me and which pointed me in the right direction. I am eternally grateful.

Amy Rhoads:
My goal with IF was to stop the weight gain, which was on an uncontrollable upward trajectory. I've already lost 20 pounds and it felt effortless. But even more importantly, my emotional binge eating had declined dramatically. My appetite control kicked in and I'm simply not tempted by the things that I used to want to eat endlessly. I crave healthier food. I get full faster. And for the first time in my 45 years, I know that I can eat what I want without feeling guilt, shame or remorse.

Now that I am eating only one meal and a snack each day, I put more thought and energy into making that food count. Instead of grabbing whatever is convenient, I put time and energy into having one satisfying meal. I try to focus on protein and vegetables because starches make me feel bloated. My husband is vegetarian but my two boys love meat, so we always have a combination of the two with each meal. After starting IF, I've learned to enjoy new things that give me the energy I need to last 24 hours. This includes quinoa, asparagus, beets, and all types of fish. I use lots of olive oil and spices. I try different cooking methods (grilling, baking, steaming, frying) to add as much flavor as possible. I've given up beef altogether as I don't feel well after I eat it. I eat all sorts of cheeses, sprinkling them on salads, in soups or as a small snack. When I have carbs, it is usually a tortilla or one piece of bread alongside tons of veggies and protein. My body seems to crave healthier food and I am able to stop eating after a much smaller amount of food. If I want something sweet, I have a cookie or a small dish of ice cream. But I no longer want to eat the entire bag of cookies or the tub of ice cream like I used to before IF.

My weight loss was very slow until I read the book (*Delay, Don't Deny*), which told me to cut diet soda and flavored sparkling water during my fasting times. You've truly convinced me that these drinks increase my insulin and prevent me from burning fat most efficiently. (My mom has been telling me this for years, but somehow, I needed your book to convince me. Sorry mom!)

K. Mikesell:

Intermittent fasting has significantly changed my relationship with self and with food. I see food as a beautiful healthy experience to enjoy respectfully. I love the freedom I have to enjoy anything that suits my fancy. I love the way that I have learned to be intuitive to my body's need to fast and need to eat. I love the respect that I am giving to my body to do what it needs to do to function better and hopefully eventually at its best. I have so much more respect for myself knowing the difference. It's been blissful. And correcting in every way.

I eat whatever I want. I have wanted whole healthy full and nourishing meals 90% of the time. And the other time is whatever suits my fancy. I crave health more and more and really can taste the processed junk these days and no longer prefer it. I love rich flavors like steaks with garlic blue cheese butter and roasted vegetables or potatoes. I enjoy desserts like berries and fresh cream and an occasional glass of wine or two.

Philip, from Jersey CI:

I've lost 2 stone in weight, which is great, but more than that, it's changed the way I think about food. I do still enjoy a takeaway, but the next day I never feel quite right. It's as if my body is more discerning. I have naturally found myself eating and genuinely enjoying healthy food choices. I've come to realise that I only ate because the clock said so or I was bored. I find it difficult to believe how easy I now find eating once a day, and even more that I now prefer black coffee to a latte: UNBELIEVABLE! Even though I haven't eaten for 24 hours, I don't feel hungry. I leave food on my plate; I never did that before. I always managed to squeeze more in. My blood pressure is now down because of the weight loss, which is great too.

I now just eat in the evening, around 8 pm. I like fresh, nutritious food that I have made myself. I love salads, with fresh leaves, tomatoes, avocado, nuts, seeds and fresh veg. I eat oily fish like sardines and salmon. I love chicken, beef and pork, and prepare them different ways. I like curries, roast dinners, stews…in fact, everything fresh.

Barb from NJ:

I just had bloodwork done and my blood sugar levels and blood pressure are great! I lost 14 lbs. in the first 10 months, and now that I am eating OMAD, I expect continued success. Gin has inspired me to keep my eating window tight and get serious.

I eat nuts and avocado daily, and no sugar. This quenches all hunger pains! From Gin's support group, I also learned to replenish with electrolytes during the fast, and that has been a big help.

144

Franki:

> I eat lots of vegetables and fruit. I eat good quality
> full-fat yoghurt. I make my own kombucha. I eat
> bread, but try and have sourdough. I make lots of
> sugar free chocolate with coconut oil and whatever
> else I fancy! It is stored in the freezer and is delicious!
>
> I have never felt freer with food. I would forbid so
> much in years gone by, where now nothing is
> forbidden. I don't eat a lot of meat but tend to prefer
> salmon, eggs, or chicken for protein. I open my
> window around 6, and depending on the day, close it
> three hours later. I do this seven days a week. I also
> drink a lot of green tea at work. At home, I drink
> coffee. IF changed my life. I haven't had a cold in
> years. I have been at goal for over 12 months.

Sarah Mallette:

> When I first started my IF journey in January of this
> year (2017), I was only concerned with weight loss. I
> "knew" fasting could be good for you, but at the time,
> didn't really know how good. Over the last almost 7
> months, I've lost 20 lbs. and a lot of inches. But the
> most important is what I GAINED! I sleep so much
> deeper. Inflammation, bloating and puffiness in my
> face have gone way down (it seemed to have
> disappeared overnight). Chronic migraines have
> gotten so much better! I've gone from 2-3 a week to
> maybe 3 a month. And even then, they're not as
> unbearable as they used to be. Food tastes amazing
> now. I no longer have depression connected to food
> issues. My skin is clear. No more constantly thinking
> about food. I still have about 40 lbs. to go to get to my
> weight loss goal, but I have no doubt that OMAD and
> IF will get me there! Even if I never lost another
> pound, I would never do anything else. I'm never
> going back!
>
> When I first started, I went a little nuts with the
> freedom. I ate junk every day. And lots of it. But
> slowly my body gravitated towards healthier foods.

Not because I had to, but because that is what my body was asking for. Vegetables of all kinds, fruit (I LOVE fruit), beans, and any and all dairy. My favorite "dessert/sweet" since I started has become vanilla Greek yogurt with strawberries and homemade whipped cream. I seriously eat anything and everything I want, though I limit processed carbs and sugar. Once again, not because I have to, but because they make me feel bad. Here's an example: I have always loved Cheetos. I could seriously eat a whole bag in one sitting (I know, I know. That's awful.) But now I can't eat them without them making me extremely sick. It's a good problem to have, trust me! I try my best to choose foods that help and nourish my body. And I'll also have the occasional Ben & Jerry's. Live your life! But be good to your body.

I hope you find as much joy and contentment with IF and OMAD as I have. I'm so thankful I stumbled onto Gin's Facebook support group, months ago, or I would still be looking for that "perfect way of eating". Thank goodness, no more searching. I've found it.

Kate from Pennsylvania:
I've lost a pound a week, on average. My energy is increased, I no longer feel bloated, I've gone down more than one dress size, and I get more compliments on my appearance now than ever before.

Whole foods make me feel best. I avoid wheat products, because they just make me gassy and bloated, but there's nothing else that I actively avoid. I eat lots of fruits and veggies, meat and seafood, nuts and seeds, sometimes wine, and I almost never skip dessert!

Walking Faster:
I am over 60, and apart from losing around 30 pounds, the best thing that has happened is a big reduction in knee pain (I am a keen hill walker and going downhill is far less painful at 64 than it was at

54). I was also getting stiffness in my hands overnight. I used to have to consciously overcome resistance and discomfort in order to curl them into fists when I woke up. I can now make tight fists fairly effortlessly. Another great gain is that I now control what I eat. As I only eat for a short time each day, I find it very easy to leave out anything I have decided is bad for me - after all, there is not really enough time on any one day to eat more than a small selection of the good stuff.

When I began fasting I was eating a strange mixture of healthy food and junk - ready meals, biscuits, crisps, sugary desserts, etc. Oddly enough, this did not stop me losing weight by fasting. But I did begin to go off them, which I could not have imagined. Then I realised I finally had the power to live off good food and not follow cravings. Because there has been diabetes and dementia in my family I decided to augment the health benefits of fasting with a no GPS diet - no grains, no potatoes, no sugars. Of course, there are no guarantees, but having seen what I have seen I am not taking any risks. Personally, I find that fasting makes restricting easier - I would find it harder to follow a plan which had forbidden foods if I had to avoid them for breakfast, lunch, dinner and snacks, but with only one meal I have more than enough delicious options to choose from without pining for what I have decided I will not have.

I am also spending the money I save from not eating all day on quality - I am finding more and more organic produce the more I look; I have started making my own milk and coconut water kefir and am introducing raw sauerkraut and raw kimchi into my diet.

Mary from Pullman:
I feel more relaxed about food and I feel more confident in myself. I went through a bad depression last winter that bordered on mental breakdown and

147

the weight loss has helped tremendously. My husband says the change is day and night!

I try to incorporate cholesterol lowering foods such as salmon, walnuts and beans, but when I go out to eat I just eat what sounds good. If I want dessert after that, then sure, why not!

OMAD has changed my life. I will continue it forever. Everyone says it scares them, and it scared me too at first, but once you get used to it, you'll see how your life can be everything you ever dreamed it would be!

Beth from New Jersey:
I have freedom from the constant thinking of food, being nervous around food and the negative self-talk I would do because of it. I am a vegan, and I feel best having the starch. It keeps me full and happy.

I have learned food is very personal. You can feel included or excluded. Opinions on what to eat and when are divided like politics.

Lillybeth in New Zealand:
IF reminds me I can 'choose' when I eat - that I don't have to be a slave to three meals a day. Also, when I make a successful lifestyle change, I become more open to doing things differently in other areas of my life too, looking at things intentionally, and with fresh eyes. Never having been worried about it before, I now buy organic from local markets/shops, free-range, etc., where possible, even though it's often more expensive. This switch isn't for my health but that of those who grow/farm the food and to be more ethical and environmentally sustainable.

I guess eating less has made me more selective, not in a food-snob way, but as a conscious consumer. The change of switching to IF has provoked more change. I'm looking at food and consumption in new light and being more selective where I spend my food dollar.

With less reliance on animal products, along with eating less in general, my shopping goes further and I end up freezing fresh foods to make them last longer, meaning I have more of a supply on-hand of good meals, rather than having to start from scratch each time I want to eat.

I'm currently eating two meals a day within a window of 5 hours, usually 1-6pm (late lunch and early dinner). I recently looked into going vegan because of the cruelty, waste and pollution caused by the industries, but decided against it as I believe we need animal-derivatives at the very least, for good health. I am seeking out vegan alternatives. My diet is currently higher in veggies / fruits / grains / beans / protein powder, low in sugar / white carbs / junk, low in animal products, (very limited dairy, no beef and only including chicken or fish every second day, aiming to be more cruelty-free in my consumption, not for health or allergy reasons).

When I first started IF, I basically ate whatever I wanted, just one meal a day. I looked a little thinner a less bloated, but realised I was still in the old habits with sugar and junk and it wasn't the freedom I wanted. Just last week I started more closely following the [a specific dietary plan's] eating style. [This plan] is carb conscious (not low carb) and includes mainly one fuel source each meal (separating fats and carbs - not lots of carbs and fats together). I'd previously had great success this way and within 1 week I can see and feel a similar improvement as I did when eating one meal of whatever I wanted. I've switched to two meals as I doubted I'd get enough protein and nutrition with less animal and dairy products and only one meal a day.

Shalini:
> I am enjoying controlled cravings, losing weight and better blood sugar levels. I eat as per my hunger, usually IF (20:4 window). I am born vegetarian and

turned vegan in Dec. 2014 to control my blood sugar levels and I got promising results. Being vegan gives me satisfaction that none of the living creatures were hurt for my meal, and it is kind of an enhanced spirituality along with super effects on health. Last but not the least, I am contributing some relief to Mother Earth by being vegan as it applies to my life style as well.

M. from St. Louis:

I am a long-term sufferer of GERD (Gastroesophageal reflux disease) or commonly known as acid reflux. Over the years I have tried everything possible from prescription medicine, as well as over the counter and holistic treatments, to no avail. I'd get better for a time and then the GERD would flare up on me again. Medicine made it worse, as it was the use of medicines to treat migraine headaches in the 80s that started this. I was about ready to resign myself this was something I'd have to live with the rest of my life. Even though eating caused excessive pain when I swallowed (feeling like someone was twisting a knife in my stomach), I still ate the 3 meals a day because I thought that was what we needed to do. I began looking at an oncoming meal with fear and dread, knowing the pain that I would have to endure for hours afterward.

Finally, I had enough and decided to look deeper into One Meal a Day, as I have done intermittent fasting in the past. I came across the book *Delay, Don't Deny*. I read the book, saw reference to the Facebook groups, and joined on May 27, 2017. In 2 weeks, by following a clean fast and eating only in my window, my GERD/acid reflux has disappeared on me and I can once again look forward to eating my one meal. I like to reference the pain I had as my stomach gathering defenses against the oncoming attack of food.

I like to open my window with something light or an ice latte made with a small drizzle of raw unfiltered honey. Anything heavy or overly sweet and I feel yucky and bloated for days. In fact, anything overly sweet and heavy anytime during my window leaves me this way for several days after.

I don't restrict what I eat but I have to restrict how much of something. I can eat fruit, but only one type of fruit at my meal. I can have a taco or a burrito but I can't eat both or I feel yucky and bloated. I do not follow any dietary restrictions and I find I do best with a 1-hour window. I started off my OMAD journey with a 4-hour window, as I was playing with 16:8 for 6 months prior, but found that 4 hours was even too long for me.

Joe O'Ski:

Intermittent Fasting helps me organize my day by freeing up wasted time preparing and eating meals my body does need. The money I saves allows me to buy the kind of food that is good for my body. I like the idea that I only need to eat once, and the rest of the hours in the day my body is healing itself, and using my fat as fuel.

I try to eat Keto because it just aligns with fasting and burning my fat, but I like the idea of being able to eat at home, or out, with any food I want, plus dessert if I want. This a way of eating that I can enjoy for a life time!

IF (Intermittent Fasting)… if you do Intermittent Fasting this year, you'll have a Happy New Rear!

Ashley Hebert:

IF has given me a new chain-less relationship with food, and therefore a new and much needed appreciation for both my internal and external body. It has freed me from the compulsive thoughts about food and allowed me to replace that time, energy, and focus with family, work, and new hobbies (the extra money and energy have been nice too!)

With IF, I try to stick to paleo eating habits with a SMALL portion of whatever else I want. That's been the magical wand for me ... instead of binging on a pack of cookies in secret because I knew I wasn't supposed to have them (rebellion is my middle name), it's actually been an easy transition for me to say, "I'll eat TWO cookies once my window opens." Making myself wait a few hours, but giving myself permission, has opened my eyes to how emotionally driven - not hunger or cravings driven - my eating had become. And by become, I mean has always been. Being a creature of rebellion and creative excuses, the black and white nature of IF has made it easy to keep my food within set timing windows, and I quickly found that once the craving-bingeing-craving-more cycle was broken, the 'bad foods' weren't what I really wanted, it was control I was after.

PCOS (Polycystic Ovary Syndrome) has robbed me (& my husband) of biological children. The same disease that drastically reduced my chances of ever being pregnant is the same one that makes me constantly look pregnant, courtesy of the constant sugar cravings and bloated stomach cycle. I've battled this cruel game for my entire adult life. Being able to conquer the physical cravings and the way my body now looks through IF (OMAD specifically) has given me power and peace.

Kat Simmons:

My body feels less painful, and my cravings and strong appetite are lessening. I've always struggled to lose weight, but this process feels natural, and as I continue to inspect and adapt my process and what works best for me in terms of IF duration, I do feel better, and if nothing else, it is worth it just for that!

I try to follow a Keto lifestyle, but noticed that I feel better with a few added carbs each week. I have started eating dairy again, but overall, I try to use good fats instead of dairy whenever possible. Occasionally, I have gluten free bread.

Kathi from California:

My rosacea has noticeably cleared, my IBS does not disrupt my life like it used to, and I feel less puffy all the time.

I eat a 90% vegan diet. When on vacation or out with friends, I'm not as strict as I am at home. I eat mostly vegetables, fruits, beans, rice, potatoes, and pasta. This keeps me satisfied during my fasting times. I don't indulge in many processed or packaged foods, but will occasionally eat them if I really have a craving. I tried the low carb, high fat thing, but I was miserable - felt sick and was always hungry. Apparently, my body is a carb-loving machine!

Lisa from New Bern, NC:

I began on January 1, 2017. I reached my goal of a 20-pound weight loss about March 10th or so. I continued IF and lost an additional 5 pounds. The way in which IF has changed my life is that I have a new relationship with food. I have always thought about what I was eating, but it was always either in diet ("being good" mode) or cheat ("being bad" mode). Now, I just have "being happy and healthy" mode as my new norm. I look up recipes that I once thought would be totally out of my range to prepare because it was way too rich, or yummy or something I deemed that made it not okay for me to make it. Now I have learned to go ahead and make it. Live life, and have it.

Being satisfied with the food I am eating takes me to a totally different place than eating the foods I didn't want in the first place, yet I ate them because some diet was telling me to eat it. No wonder I'd binge. Now I eat salad with full strength dressing, cheese and avocado because I like the way all those things taste together. Hey, add the croutons and bacon! I love to taste test while I am cooking, just like they do on TV. I have a snack when I come home to break my fast, and then I start making dinner for my family. I often end with a treat. It might be sweet, but it might be some chips if it goes with my meal. Sometimes I have seconds of a meal, but I no longer feel the need to over eat. Food has become my good friend. I carefully think about how I want to prepare things now.

I want to eat healthier because I am feeling the effects of good food. I also gave up soda, lots of processed foods, and I have learned to read labels. I save so much money eating less! I not only now buy better foods, but going out to restaurants has lost much of it appeal because, to be honest, I can usually cook it better, and plus I know what's in it. My kids are eating better as well. They have favorite recipes now.

I make desserts on Sunday afternoons these days, just like I did as a kid. I love establishing traditions and memories. Food has become a lifelong friend instead of a foe. My favorite foods now sit happily in the middle of the table, waiting to be enjoyed, instead of hiding, stashed away in the dark corners of the cabinet.

I find I am trying recipes with lots of new ingredients. Leeks, almonds, avocados, garlic, dark chocolate, barley, soy beans, kale and olive oil have all been new food additions. I absolutely love my air fryer! It gets all the unnecessary oils and other yuckos out of it before I eat it. I now get crunchy texture without all the added oils. I have definitely become much more aware of what I am consuming. If I eat too much, I usually have to lay down. Naps do me wonders. I often feel re-energized and not hungry! Fasting helps me mentally prepare for the food I am about to enjoy. Health benefits are fabulous as well.

I started IF Jan. 1, 2017 and reached my first goal about March 10. I continued this way of eating, lost a few more pounds, and reached a new all-time low of 124 lbs. Never did I think I could get here. I have been here now for months. IF has allowed me a maintenance program that works! I consider this my new base weight. I do check in on the scale periodically but I no longer feel chained to it. I no longer giving this silly piece of metal the authority to make or break my day. I found I lost the most weight when I put the scale away for a while. I would challenge myself to not weigh for a week or so and then I was often happily surprised.

Rachel from Florida:

IF has given me the power to free myself from calorie counting and take control of my hunger. Calorie counting worked for a while, but then it stopped, and I found myself hungry all the time. I also felt like when I obsessed about ingredients in my food, it made it difficult to go out with friends and turned me into a hermit. With IF I don't have to stress so much about WHAT I'm eating, just when I'm eating. I have stopped weighing myself, so I only go by the size of my pants, but I have definitely dropped a couple of pant sizes. But more importantly, I've taken control of my hunger and did away with the mindless snacking. Plus, it is very freeing to go many hours without food and remind yourself that you're not going to die.

As of right now I don't restrict myself too much, because I come from a very restrictive background. As far as time goes, early dinner time works best for me I've found. I also make sure to drink a lot of tea during my fasting period because I love it. I do avoid soda as much as possible, though, as I do not feel that has a healthy place in my diet. And whenever eating I try my best to get nutritious vegetables. My favorite meals at home are usually hearty salads.

Martha Gonzalez:
>Yes, I have had weight loss, but also no more migraines, no more leg spasms at night, no more fatigue, no more heartburn, and numerous other conditions that I no longer experience.

>I find that when I eat burgers or processed foods I get migraines as soon as I eat...so I try to eat as clean as possible.

Missy from Texas:
>Control. Results. Discipline. Freedom.

>I eat in a 2-4 hour window, 5 to 7 days per week. Sometimes I open my window longer on the weekends to allow for more social experiences with my family and friends. While I am in no way on a ketogenic diet, I actually prefer a high protein, low carbohydrate diet. My body actually responds very well to this for my overall health—I have a history of rheumatoid arthritis, ankylosing spondylitis and severe allergies.

>What I love MOST about OMAD, is that I CAN have whatever I want. With previous attempts at a low carb diet, I missed fruit desperately. I still like some bread/bread products on occasion but I do not crave them. I love the sense of freedom with OMAD.

>I am active. I feel healthy. I have dropped from 162 to 146 (best all-time low--let's be realistic, it fluctuates), but I am thinner, my clothes fit better, and I feel better about myself in general.

Ursula from Augusta:
>Intermittent fasting has taken me off the rollercoaster of food addiction. It has stopped my constant pre-occupation with food (what will I eat next; will it help me to lose weight?) I feel like I have been set free!

Right now, I'm eating low carb, with no sugar or artificial sweeteners. By eating low carb, it keeps the swelling of my legs down, and it keeps me from retaining excess fluids.

I absolutely love the huge amount of energy I have since doing intermittent fasting. I feel so much better and I'm moving so much better My constant hunger monster is finally under control.

Sarah Samuel:
I have gone from my highest weight of 175-ish lbs. to 162 lbs. in just 2.5 months, eating pretty much whatever I want. The weight loss is AWESOME, but what's even better is that I just don't get hungry as much as I used to. If you had told me five months ago to fast regularly for 19 hours a day, sometimes up to 22 hours, I would tell you it was impossible! And now I do it without any trouble. When I do get hungry, it no longer feels like an emergency, which allows me some calm and peace around food and eating, and I hardly ever get hungry until right before I'm going to eat.

The other thing that's been awesome is I don't feel guilty anymore when I eat junk food, and I'm much more in touch with what my body wants to eat, which are the foods my mind is slowly starting to want to eat too, like salads and green smoothies. I finally feel like I'm truly fueling my body instead of just eating out of old habits and comfort.

My food tastes are extremely varied, so to keep it short, I want to talk about two of my favorite foods that I eat multiple times a week: bagels & chia seed pudding. The great thing about IF is that I can eat whatever I want, and I pretty much always want to eat a bagel, so that's a staple of my diet. I think the fat from the avocado, eggs, and cream cheese that I eat with it help me to not feel that bloated carby feeling after eating one.

The other great thing about IF is that since I'm only eating one or two meals a day, and because I know that my goal is to reduce my insulin levels, heal my probably fatty liver, and give my body the nutrients it needs to function properly, I have to really prioritize healthy food like salads and green smoothies. One of my favorite meals to prioritize is chia seed pudding! I make a big batch of it with just the water and chia seeds, and then each day when I eat it, I add full fat Greek yogurt (vegan yogurt is great too, or omit the yogurt!), almond butter, cinnamon, fruit, and pumpkin seeds. Nuts, coconut flakes, coconut oil, and hemp seeds are also great additions! This meal is so satiating and delicious, and gives me tons of energy, without making me feel full and lethargic. In general, I feel best when I eat mostly plants (though I love eggs and like to indulge in cheese and fish every once in awhile), and when I get enough fiber and fat.

Lisa, the Crunchy Midwife:

As of this writing, I've lost roughly 12 pounds in a month's time and (forgive me for saying!), I'm looking good!! I have a long way to go yet, but the feeling of looser clothes and looking thinner, as I see myself in the mirror, has a way of boosting self-esteem like nobody's business! The fact that I can pull this off without feeling deprived is huge, but what's more exciting is that I know IF is sustainable, unlike so many other ways that I've attempted to lose weight in the past. Feeling good about yourself is the BEST feeling evah!

My first week, I truly ate whatever I wanted during my 2-hour eating window and dropped a good amount of weight. As my body acclimates, I've found that I'm not interested in wasting my window on things that fill but don't satisfy. I lean towards ketogenic style eating because I've really messed up my metabolism over the years with low calorie diets. I want to support my body's intention to right some wrongs. If I eat simple carbs, I feel yucky and bloated. Veggies make my body happy and I feel energetic when I eat a rainbow of colors. Good fats like avocado and walnuts keep me super satisfied and proteins like salmon, grass fed beef and pastured chicken help me fill full, which I like. Yep! I said it. I LIKE feeling full and satisfied!! No "diet" has ever done that for me y'know?

Thanks Gin for being a light bearer in the world of IF.

Belle from PA:
I just finished my second week, and I reached a weight that I haven't been in 3 years!!! I also have more energy for my fasted workouts than I have unfasted, and my sleep is sooo solid! I'm really feeling great!!!

I eat LCHF (low carb high fat) and NSNG (no sugar no grains). I enjoy a large variety of vegetables, protein in the form of eggs, fish, and chicken, healthy fats like nuts, avocado, cheese, and grass-fed butter, with wine on occasion.

Gail from Pittsburgh:
IF has given me so much freedom. I used to have to eat at least three meals a day once I started eating, and since I eat primarily meat and vegetables, I had to cook three times a day as well. That ate up a lot of my day. I was terrified to go too long without eating due to reactive hypoglycemia. I could end up with low blood sugar, nausea, cold sweats, extreme hunger, and even passing out. Due to IF, that no longer happens. I also get a lot more done during the day.

My day is no longer ruled by wondering and planning what I am going to do about food. When I maintain my "no sugar" way of eating with IF, I also have boundless energy, much more so than I had while eating low carb. I am also a carboholic. I love carbs, or at least my taste buds do, but my body does not. With IF, I have been able to fit in a few carbs from time to time without throwing myself completely out of whack. I have also overindulged, but have not gained the 10 - 15 pounds that might normally get packed on. I have gained no more than 4 pounds and I put that totally to the IF.

LCHP (low carb, high protein) makes me feel my best. This has been a long journey over many years. I followed all different kinds of diets over the years trying to keep my weight and appetite under control. I had also developed some health problems, such as chronic fatigue, IBS, hypoglycemia, and hypothyroidism. Over time, I found that by eating animal proteins and low carb vegetables, I felt much better. I do not do well with rendered fats. I use olive oil and butter for any extra fat that is not in my foods. I am very sensitive to sugars and can only eat a slice of fruit or a few berries with impunity. IF, however, has meant that if I eat them right before my window closes, I don't have as many side effects. I do not eat whole grains at all. I can get away with eating white flour products very intermittently; overindulgence results in all of my symptoms reemerging.

Krystal Guillory:
I had lost 26 lbs. before starting IF by eating low carbs and exercising, but that took about 9 months. While it was exciting, it seemed arduous and slow. I am a Type 2 diabetic and some days my sugar would drop or rise so much to the point of me having cold sweats and feeling like I would pass out. I started IF at the suggestion of my husband. I was very leery of this plan, as I couldn't fathom not eating for such a long period and having stable sugar levels.

I started 1 month and 3 days ago, and I have lost 10 lbs. I have so many NSVs (non-scale victories), such as my wedding ring fitting for the first time in ten years, my clothes falling off, not getting winded when taking the stairs, having tons of energy during the day, and never feeling shaky or nauseous because my sugar is too low or high. I have also cut my metformin prescription in half, and I'm hoping to completely eliminate it in the future.

I pretty much follow the DDD (*Delay, Don't Deny*) mentality. Because I do have a lot more weight to lose, I do watch my carbs at times and try to make healthier choices; but I'm more drawn to healthy choices now for my carbs. For instance, I would choose zucchini and lentil pasta as my carbs over candy bars, etc. Now, I do indulge, too. The other day my body really wanted some ice cream, so I got a small shake from Chick-fil-A. I truly couldn't drink a third of it. My body was satisfied with just a little bit: it wanted the chicken nuggets! My son gladly finished the shake for me!

As for how and when I eat, I follow IF 7 days a week, but my window fluctuates. The longest eating window is 8 hours, but I find I don't lose much with that large of a window. I typically do 20/4-- sometimes a little less or a little longer. I definitely do OMAD (one meal a day).

I typically open my window with a snack (goldfish crackers and a veggie pack, a pickle, or a small portion of protein) and my favorite beverage (1/3 sweet tea with peach from Sonic). Then I'll eat dinner with my family and perhaps a snack or fruit before bed. I haven't changed our dinners: we eat tacos, spaghetti, pork roast, pizza, etc. I do try to include a veggie each night, and now we make our own pizza. Not eating breakfast has allowed me to sleep later and not feel so rushed in the morning. Because I do clean fasting, I drink a lot of water. My skin is definitely glowing with all the water. I love not having to plan tons of snacks or check my sugar, etc.!

Wanda Baynham:

I overheard my coworker talking about *Delay, Don't Deny*. Immediately, I wanted to know more and was directed to our school's Assistant Principal. After a briefing me on the "DDD" philosophy, she let me borrow her book that day. Eagerly, I read each page, and then began reading it out loud to my precious husband. On Thursday, March 23, 2017, I borrowed the book that I finished reading Saturday morning, March 25, 2017. Those dates are important because that Saturday became the first day of a healthier way of living! Never again will we be controlled by food!

At the closing months of 2016, my husband was 49 lbs. heavier, and I was 37 lbs. heavier than our weight today. We look leaner and feel better than we have in years! My husband came home after his check up and shared some wonderful news this past July! Not only had he lost weight since January, his A1C had dropped from 7.3 to 5.5! His doctor told him to keep doing what he was doing!

When people ask me what I do if I become hungry, I tell them. Fasting reminds me to lay those precious people who have NOTHING to eat, who are sick, homeless, lost, depressed, etc. at the feet of Jesus Christ in prayer. Intermittent Fasting reminds me that I am blessed and should never take anything for granted. So, as I enjoy drinking clean water and black coffee, I pray for others that I do not know. My walk with my Heavenly Father is even sweeter than it was six months ago, because I have even more time with Him. I am thankful that he used Gin, an unselfish person, willing to share the TRUTH about what worked in her life through her book, *Delay, Don't Deny*!

As of today, our fasting average (Hubby and me) is about 19 hours a day. That totally depends on our day, though. Freedom to adjust is WONDERFUL AND GUILTLESS! The majority of our food choices are organic, which makes us feel the best. We will choose to eat junk occasionally and suffer the bloating afterwards! Food choices have changed as we look for QUALITY in what we eat! My husband is a diabetic, and continues to monitor his blood sugar. He will eat a real piece of cake, not made with artificial sweeteners. We no longer use them (artificial sweeteners), but still use common sense and don't eat (nor desire to eat) dessert every day!

Susan from B.C.:

Since starting IF, I have found my power. I'm a much stronger person! I never thought I would be able to go for 20 hours a day without any food and enjoy it.

I see so many changes. Before I started, I was 210 lbs. and busting out of a size 16. I couldn't go up a flight of stairs without concentration, because I was always concerned my knees would give out, due to osteo-arthritis. I was always tired and lacked a desire to do anything. Now I've been fasting for just over 2 months and I have so much energy. My arthritis is almost non-existent. I love walking and hiking, and I can go up the stairs without even holding the hand rail. I have been on 200 mg of Levothyroxine for almost 30 yrs. I have now had that cut in half and I feel great. Over the years I've had my meds cut but they always end up raising them again. This is the second blood test and I'm still doing great on the 1/2 dose. I have lost 19 lbs. and have gone down 3 pant sizes. My doctor is very impressed with my weight loss and sees all the benefits.

I love all food… I have a soy allergy so I make it all myself. If I ever eat out I am prepared for my allergy. I fast until 3 pm and open my 4-hour window with a banana and nuts, or avocado and tomatoes. Something light and easy on the stomach. Then I relax for about an hour, after which I will prepare my main meal. I try my best to eat resistant starches, including carbs that are cooked one day and cooled till the next,

163

then reheated to eat. They change the chemistry for great health benefits like healing my gut. I have one plate of food, but eat till just full. Some days that means I get a bit more. Other days it means I can't finish my serving. Usually dinner is a small amount of chicken or fish, a good portion of resistant starch, and veggies. I enjoy a salad. Sometimes I'll make pasta and serve it lots of ways. I don't eat soy or red meat, but everything else is fair game. With one meal a day, it's a feast.

I know I'm healing from within. I see my eczema gone, my energy is restored, and I sleep very well. When I fast, I fast clean. This means I wake to black coffee (approximately 3 cups at breakfast). The rest of my day I drink filtered water or sparkling water. Always plain, no flavours. I don't want to spike my insulin and break my fast. Most mornings I go for a walk and exercise. I'm living my life much better than before IF.

Being a part of Gin's IF group has been a game changer for me. It is a lifestyle and the longer I do it the easier it gets.

Australian Intermittent Faster:
I have always been fairly thin but struggled to lose baby weight after each baby. After my third I reached a point where I realised I really needed to do something, so I started going to the gym and really restricting what I ate. In hindsight, I was skipping meals: I would have a meal replacement shake for breakfast, a few carrots and celery for lunch, then a full normal dinner with my family. Then my husband was asked to move overseas for work. It was a stressful decision initially, but once I found my feet I made great friends and enjoyed my time there. Every day was like a holiday (do I need to eat that big plate of poutine? No, but eat it now and worry about it when you move back home). The move was life changing for me in many ways though. My husband,

unbeknownst to anyone but me, was abusive, and I finally found the courage to leave him. The divorce was stressful, but I was really happy. However, by this stage, and in my early 40s, I had developed a form of bulimia. So those times I was out with friends, eating like I was on a 2-week holiday, I would come home afterwards and force myself to vomit. This continued for about 2 years. I kidded myself that because I was only purging once every few weeks, that it wasn't really bulimia. In hindsight, I don't think it was, but it was certainly some type of eating disorder. The absolute lowest point was driving from Buffalo airport en route to home, and eating breakfast with my girls in McDonald's, then vomiting afterwards in the dirty washroom there.

After 4 years, I decided to move back home to Australia, and by this stage I was carrying 10-15 extra kilos. I had promised myself that I would view this move as a fresh start and not purge anymore. For the most part I was successful, but by this stage I think I had destroyed my metabolism and I found it very hard to shift those last kilos. I tried my faithful shakes but with no success. I then tried [a diet company's products]. It worked, but I put the weight back on.

From there, I stumbled upon 5:2 intermittent fasting, then on a Facebook page someone mentioned clean fasting. I read *Delay, Don't Deny*, and *The Obesity Code*, and realised that when I thought I was fasting, I really wasn't.

I am very, very slowly losing the last of my 'holiday' weight, and just this morning experienced my first whoosh. But the best part for me is I have absolutely no desire to go back to my bad eating disorder habits. I fast, then I feast. And I feel no guilt at all during the feasting. I eat until I'm full. And I really have never felt better, inside and out.

I have an Italian background so the idea of not eating pasta does not work. I really do eat whatever I want. I cook homemade meals for my girls so we tend not to eat takeaway a lot. At home I'll cook Italian meals, stir fries, and we also eat a lot of sushi.

I have realised during this journey that I am a social and emotional eater. So, while I'm not hungry while fasting, I initially mourned the loss of the social aspect of eating at work. I've learned to be happy sitting with a tea or coffee with my co-workers instead. If I'm having a stressful day, I no longer feed my stress at lunch on sweets and chocolate. So, in a sense, IF also forces you to find other ways to deal with stress. Healthier ways.

Susan Zamzow:

Can I just say, I feel so darn happy, inside and out! I feel at peace with food.

I used to eat pretty low carb, writing down everything I ate, and counting every calorie. However, I wasn't losing the weight. I chalked it up to my hypothyroidism. Then I found Gin on Facebook, and my life turned upside down.

I no longer count calories, or deprive myself of carbs. I still do my best to choose clean, whole foods, but if I really want something, I have it. I no longer deny myself. I do know that I feel most satisfied when I eat more veggies and lean meats, and cut back on pastas and breads. However, if I am really wanting a particular food, I have it (in my eating window of course).

I am currently down 20 pounds in 5 months. I have 10 to go, but I no longer stress over it. It will come off eventually. What's most important now is that I feel freed from the "diet" rollercoaster. My insides feel so good, with no bloating, or uncomfortable feelings.